I0698743

VITAMINS & SUPPLEMENTS CAN BENEFIT YOU!

25 Common Health Conditions Examined

Frank C Auenson

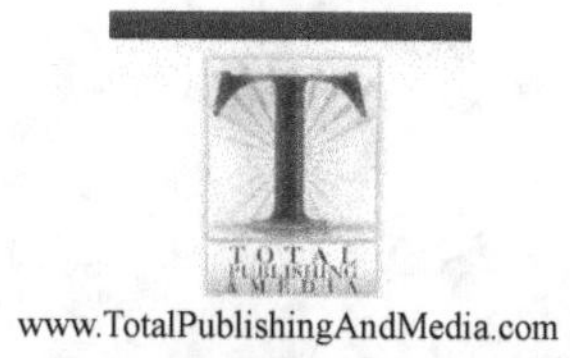

www.TotalPublishingAndMedia.com

© Copyright 2023, Frank C Auenson

All rights reserved.

No part of this book may be reproduced, stored in a
retrieval system, or transmitted by any means,
electronic, mechanical, photocopying, recording,
or otherwise, without written permission
from the author.

ISBN: 978-1-63302-255-3

I now know my father knew what he was talking about
regarding all the supplements he took in his 80s/90s!
Thank you, Dad!

FOREWORD

In today's world we have access to a great deal of information. There are numerous vitamins and supplements on the market today, how do you know what is right for you? Or for that matter what ails you?

Have you ever considered how great it would be to have information about the top ailments that affect hundreds of thousands of people and natural ways to overcome these issues at your fingertips? Now you have that ability. Frank Auenson has done extensive research to make this possible for those that choose to take the time to read this book.

I know firsthand that the supplements work. I was having trouble focusing on conversations and being able to recall words. If you have never experienced this, you may not realize how troubling it is. It is frightening. I began taking Neuro Up and within a couple of weeks my focus began getting better, I was able to recall words and carry-on conversations with ease. There are medications on the market to help with mental clarity however why would I want to put chemicals in my body when there is a natural solution. I don't.

I have had the pleasure of working with Frank and know the commitment he has made to providing you with pertinent information about each ailment and each vitamin. As a certified nutritionist, I can tell you that the information provided in this book is accurate.

However, it is always important to contact your physician before starting any vitamin or supplements.

Frank writes in an easy, straightforward manner which allows you to easily understand what the vitamins do to help your body. I encourage you to read this book and find out how vitamins and supplements can help you!

~ Debbie Goodman, ISSA Certified Nutritionist

TABLE OF CONTENT

Chapter Summaries

Chapter 1. Many people have allergies, the important thing is to not ignore symptoms and consult your physician if you notice anything unusual. Consider alternative natural ways to ease symptoms.

Chapter 2. We have all dealt with anxiety in our lives. But if you find that it is a constant factor, consider natural remedies.

Chapter 3. Arthritis can affect most of us as our bodies age. Much like how our everyday items show wear and tear, joints are no different.

Chapter 4. There are multiple types of cancers that can strike anyone at any age at any time. Be mindful of how your body feels and looks and if anything seems different from the norm, consult your doctor.

Chapter 5. If you're constantly feeling tired and/or depressed, consult your doctor. You are not alone and there are people and products that can help.

Chapter 6. CAD is most likely to happen as we hit our middle to later years. Diet, exercise, restful sleep, and medications can help lower your blood pressure.

Chapter 7. Suck it up buttercup doesn't exactly work when it comes to depression. Medication is usually over-prescribed to help, but side effects are common. Learn about what treatments are available that are right for you, including alternates like vitamins and other supplements.

Chapter 8. Diabetes is a high risk for those in the U.S. Due to high levels of sugar in most everything along with a sedentary lifestyle. There are medications that can help, but diet and exercise are the biggest factors here.

Chapter 9. ED can be caused by many things and can affect all men. Do not fret, consult your doctor on suggestions for life changes or supplements that could help.

Chapter 10. Fibromyalgia is not only brought on by physical conditions, but mental ones as well. There are many over the counter vitamins that could help with this.

Chapter 11. Headaches affect many people. Rest is the best treatment. However, if headaches don't go away after a couple of days or get worse, consult your physician.

Chapter 12. Hypertension is starting to affect more people day by day, not only diet but the constant stress of our daily lives. Consult your doctor on the best way to handle it.

Chapter 13. High Cholesterol is commonly caused by unhealthy foods and a sedentary lifestyle. Exercise, better diets and some medications are first considered the best way to deal with it.

Chapter 14. Menopause affects all women eventually. Consult your physician for any vitamins or procedures to reduce symptom discomfort.

Chapter 15. Multiple Sclerosis is a disease that can hinder the body's ability to do what most of us would consider the easiest things. One would almost believe that the body is turning against itself.

Chapter 16. Obesity is a rising concern in the U.S. High calorie intake and fatty foods along with a sedentary lifestyle can cause weight gain at an alarming rate. Diet changes and exercise are the most reliable ways to combat it.

Chapter 17. Peripheral Neuropathy can start with the hands and/ or feet, with numbness or tingling. It can progress up the arms and legs as well. Different forms of therapy along with some vitamins and medications can help to lessen the effects.

Chapter 18. Plantar fasciitis is the pain that starts on the bottom of the heel and can move to the arch of the foot. Proper shoes or inserts can help along with physical therapy and medications to help with pain and inflammation.

Chapter 19. Psoriasis is when the body produces too many skin cells in a certain area, causing it to dry out and rise up as patches on the body. Learn the difference between Psoriasis and a simple rash.

Chapter 20. Post-Traumatic Stress Disorder is the mind re-living a traumatic or extreme emotional event from our lives. Consult your doctor or therapist for *the* option that's best for you.

Chapter 21. Restless Leg Syndrome effects your legs with various forms of stimuli that can vary in severity, from something crawling along your leg to aches, itching, etc.

Chapter 22. Shingles is a painful rash that normally forms around the abdomen, caused by the chickenpox virus. Consult your doctor for the remedy best for you.

Chapter 23. Sleep Apnea is your body constantly stopping and starting breathing throughout your sleep cycle. A CPAP machine is usually prescribed to help after a sleep study is performed.

Chapter 24. Tendinitis the inflammation of a tendon that attaches to the bone. Normally, the knee or elbow. Rest, ice and stretching are normal forms of recovery.

Chapter 25. Tinnitus is the ringing in your ear. Normally caused by constant exposure to loud noises. But can also be from earwax build up and water in the ear.

Chapter 26. Thyroid Disease can have a couple of different effects on your body. Causing your metabolism to speed up or having your metabolism slow way down. Both can have serious effects on your body.

My Story

My name is Frank Auenson, author and now CEO/owner of Stand Alone Fitness, llc, While I am just an average guy, going through life with the ups and downs like millions of others, a chain of events made my life so much more. This led to me wanting to inspire and improve, not only my life but the lives of as many people as I could. My hope is that you will be inspired…….

My story began a few years ago when I was 40 pounds overweight and went through triple bypass surgery and a ruptured appendix at the same time. To hear this story, you would be amazed by the adventures I went through. Yes, I said adventures.

Months prior to these adventures, my doctors were concerned about my high blood pressure and felt I needed to have a stress test. Even though I knew carrying an extra 40 pounds wouldn't be pretty, I gave in and said yes.

As you can imagine, it went as I expected. I almost got to level 4 before I had had enough. Call it boredom or perhaps just done running on a treadmill but I didn't want to go on. Of course, the tape showed something yet not enough to warrant having a cardiologist come in or having to go to the emergency room.

As soon as I got home, there were phone calls from the doctor, putting me on meds and scheduling an appointment with a cardiologist.

Fun times were on the horizon as I sat down with the doctor. He began telling me how unreliable the stress test was and we could try a few more tests to see exactly what was going on. You know the deal, one test just a little more reliable than the next and so on.

Knowing the kind of guy I am, I am not one to dilly dally, let's get to the ultimate procedure that will tell us exactly what we need to know. As much of an inconvenience as it was, I went in for a heart catheterization, where they run a line with a camera up through the wrist and into the arteries of the heart.

Of course, it didn't go without complications as I was supposed to be under during the procedure. In the corner on my eye, I could see the wire in my body on the monitor and all of a sudden, my head got really hot where I even asked, "is my head supposed to get this hot?" They look over at me and instantly swing into action. I don't remember what happened after that until I was told I had two partial blockages where stents could have been placed but the stent doctor doing the procedure was uncomfortable doing so because the partial blockages were where one of my arteries forked.

He was concerned a stent would cause other issues, so he backed out to give me the wonderful news. You got it, heart surgery.

Loved the meeting with my heart surgeon. Yes, at first it was a bit of stereotyping as he was a renowned heart surgeon from Japan and while it was difficult to understand him, we had common ground, my heart.

He proceeded to show the film of my heart catheterization and point out the area of most concern. Of course, we decided a bypass surgery was the course of action needed but wait a minute, we have another area of concern as well.

Yes, another artery had a partial blockage of 60%, had it been 50%, they wouldn't have worry about it but since it's 60% they have to mention it.

I have no idea what the difference between 50% and 60% is other than 10% but I guess it was the benchmark where they determined it wouldn't hinder my life or it could potentially be a problem down the road.

And you guessed it, my heart surgeon wasn't a stent doctor. I would have to go through another heart catheterization to have a stent placed in that area of concern and believe me, it wasn't any kind of picnic the first time around so I was like, "what do you suggest doctor?"

His response and my thoughts were where magic happened. He mentioned it would only take about 15-20 minutes to do another bypass and right away I was like, well you have me there, I am wide open and certainly not going anywhere, might as well take care of it.

So that was the plan, date set and something to look forward to, right? But wait, what could possibly hinder heart surgery? Perhaps elevated white cell count with no explanation of why?

Okay Frank, you need to go see your doctor. It might surprise you that while during this appointment, I wasn't so forthcoming to get to the quick answer. Nope, they wanted to send me to the ER right then and I was having none of that.

They scheduled a CT scan for the next morning which was more to my liking. CT scan comes and goes and as soon as I get home, I get a phone call from my doctor's nurse, "you need to get to the ER as soon as possible, you have a ruptured appendix". "Oh wonderful!" I reply.

I knew I hadn't felt good the previous couple weeks but thought it was simply some sort of flu bug I was getting over. Had no idea I was walking around with a huge abscess of yuck in my gut.

Yes, I could have and should have died from this according to the medical world.

Crazy to say the least, I get my son to take me to the ER where everyone is happy to see me, right? Nope, not after reading my medical records and seeing I was scheduled for heart surgery.

Here is what usually happens to someone with a ruptured appendix, they remove your appendix and clean out your abdominal cavity of all the infectious pus that collects in the abdomen. Nice picture huh? Again, yuck! So, what happened to me?

Everything stopped!

A wonderful ER doctor comes in and wants to show me the results of the CT scan.

"You see this big black hole in the middle? It's not supposed to be there! Yet, with your pending heart surgery, we are still trying to figure out the course of action. A patient who is scheduled for heart surgery must have a weak heart so we can't operate on him."

Yes, that was the reaction.

Yet, they had to get antibiotics in me to cure the infection and take care of the big black hole in my gut. I am just telling you what the x-rays showed. Or was it a cloud?

As it turns out, I spent six days in the hospital as they had inserted a drain into my side to drain the infectious gunk and this was the course of action for the next 4 weeks with regular check-ups.

I love those Frankenstein lab looking procedure rooms. Not!

The funny thing is, during my hospital visit, my heart surgeon came to visit me and he assured me, I was in no imminent danger regarding my heart. He knew it, I knew it, but all those other doctors didn't know it.

Thank goodness it went down the way it did because from the general surgeon's reaction, I could have been strapped with a colostomy bag and this annoying drain was bad enough.

While I thought I was too young to be pooping in a bag on my side, there was a resident surgeon who was chomping at the bit to get me into the OR room. Yikes!

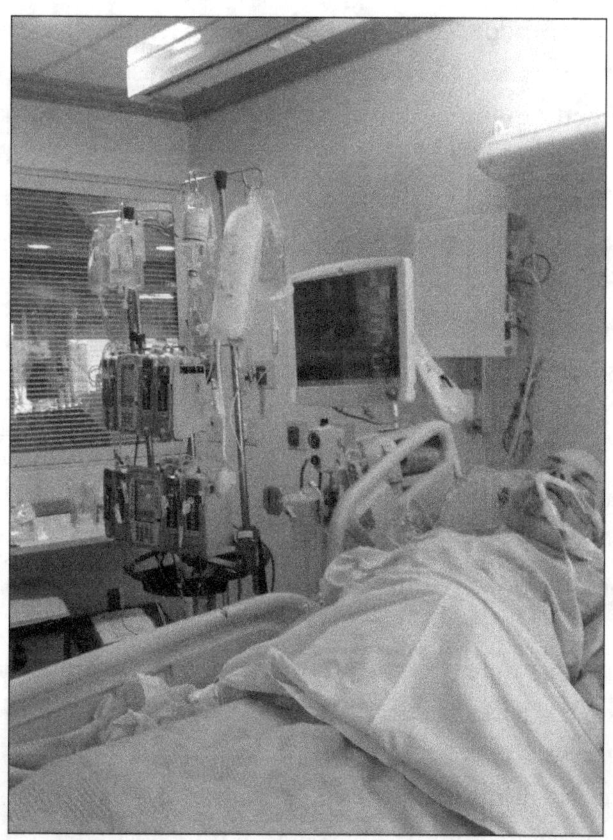

The heart surgery occurred a month later and went like clock-work. Within 24 hours, I was strolling laps around the nurse's station.

I mean literally. 3 ½ days after heart surgery, I was released and restricted to sleeping on my back for 3 months. Oh joy!

It was an agonizing recovery. Well, not really. Sure, there were things I couldn't do like sleep on my side, lift anything with any real weight. Heck, even a gallon of milk was questionable in my eyes.

I was terrified with everything I did. I mean, I had my chest cracked in two and had arteries cut from my body to replace the arteries which were clogged. I have no idea how the replacements actually stayed in place and was worried I would spring a leak.

The biggest concern was the 12-week healing process where they didn't want me doing certain things because the doctors didn't want me getting a bone infection in my chest. I guess that would have been bad news and an intense recovery in itself. No thanks!

And being a guy, I wanted to know how long it would be before I could have sex. Again, I am a guy and it's how we gage our recovery. I was told four weeks. Whew, it would be tough but I could live with that.

I was told I needed to get out walking several times a day to exercise my heart. So, I would bundle myself up and go for a walk, by myself. I walked slowly at first and I am sure some neighbors wondered who that old guy was walking like he needed a walker.

I was wearing an old man flannel jacket and a hat so I know how I looked. It was comfortable and to tell you the truth, I was sick so I didn't care what others thought.

During this time, I lost weight but I lost the weight that makes you look sick and instead of finding a way to adjust the look, I instead, gained the weight back and then some.

One day, I went for a walk, got half a mile into my usual mile walk and I was feeling like garbage in my chest area. I would rub my chest and stretch my left shoulder/arm area and wonder what was going on. Was I having a heart attack?

How could that be? I thought they fixed my heart. What kind of quality of life was I going to have if I felt like this now at my age? I was concerned but I was also mad. My heart surgeon said I wouldn't have any more issues for at least 25 years and by then, I wouldn't care.

But I did care! I didn't want to feel like this nor did I want to be a burden to anyone I had already counted on to get me through all of this. I was getting furious, what was going on? Why was I feeling so crummy?

I happened to have a chance meeting with a neighbor who years ago, had had quadruple bypass surgery. I told him what had happened and how frightened I was, thinking they had fixed my heart.

He asked me what medications I was on and I told him. "That's where the problem is, Frank. They fixed your heart alright, but the medications you are on are fighting your activity. The cardiologist tells you to exercise and work your heart but then prescribes medications that are intended to keep your heart calm and beating at a low rate."

He went on to tell me "it took over 2 years before they finally adjusted my meds where I felt somewhat normal."

Somewhat normal? Sorry but that wasn't going to work for me. If it is the meds that are causing the discomfort, something needed to change. Then I remember my doctor telling me, if I lost 25 pounds, he would take me off the 3 medications he had me on.

I was like, how am I supposed to lose 25 pounds and get off the meds if the meds are fighting my activity and especially exercising? I didn't like taking the meds but I felt I had to be a good soldier and do what they told me. I mean, they know best about this right?

There had to be another way.

Again, I needed to be able to exercise to lose the weight but not be hampered by the meds. I didn't like that feeling at all and then I took charge. It's my body, I am going to put in it what I feel is right and stop taking what was causing me issues.

Yet, I still needed to lose the weight and consume things that would be good for my heart. I mean, I have a lot to do so I need to live a good long life, right? Just the same, I wanted to be happy and feel healthy.

It took the longest time for me to understand how my heart was fixed but due to the bypass surgery, I would always be considered to have a bad heart. Never had a heart attack which means no damage but now I had to be conscious of it.

When I would exercise, such as ride a bike around the block, I knew my heart was fixed by the shortness of the recovery time. Maybe 30 second to a minute and that was a good thing.

I eventually biked around the conservancy near me (3.65 miles from driveway to driveway) for the first time and thought when I was finished, I was going to die. My heart was pounding so hard but then after about a minute, I was completely back to normal.

By the end of the summer last year, I was riding the 3.65 miles in less than 20 minutes and making the nearby hills like a champ. It was a great feeling.

So, what changed?

Since my bypass surgery and the removal of the drain, I have also done a lot of research, hundreds of hours easily. I was researching how with age, our bodies change (yes, I am 59 years old) and the imbalances we experience.

I realized, going to the gym did nothing for me and/or my weight loss struggles.

There was nothing at the gym that I couldn't do on my own, with my own resources and in my own environment. Yet, there was more to it. Yes, remember the imbalances I mentioned.

While I had taken myself off the medication prescribed and feeling better, I was still looking for my natural remedies to correcting my imbalances and in doing so, I started researching and investigating in vitamins and natural supplements.

I needed to know what vitamins I was lacking and how to replenish what my body needed. I needed to learn more about the supplement industry and how I could benefit from it.

I lost weight during my ordeal but with gaining the weight back, I wanted to help myself naturally to lose the weight again and be where I needed to be.

I still have a ways to go to reach the goals I desire but just the same, I was so impressed with my discoveries and the solutions to my imbalances, that I created **Stand Alone Fitness, llc**, the company credited with changing my life forever!

What is this new company you might be asking yourself and what were the discoveries that I found that *have* the abilities to make life changing transformations?

I began to figure out what hormones my body was starting to produce less of and what vitamins and minerals I was deficient in. It was this discovery that brought me to create **Stand Alone Fitness**, a vitamins and supplements company. Yet, there is so much more.

I knew I wanted to help others who were feeling sluggish and also struggling with their weight and/or other areas of their lives.

I wanted to show them that they were not alone in their struggles and that there were ways and products available to them to have the desired look, feel and happiness they sought after.

Did you know, according to the most recent *US Dietary Guidelines*, a record number of Americans aren't getting sufficient amounts of dietary fiber, potassium, choline, magnesium, calcium, iron, and vitamins, A, D, E, and C?

So, what do we do when we have one or more nutritional deficiencies? We either tweak our food choices or take supplements to fill the gaps.

In fact, 86% of Americans take some sort of vitamins or supplements to enhance their lifestyle. 68% of those Americans that take a vitamin or supplement are over 60 years old. Right around the corner for me.

As I mentioned earlier, I don't like going to gyms, nothing against them as they serve a purpose for others in one way or another but just not for me. I am a lone-wolf sort of person so a company like Stand Alone Fitness resonates with me.

Besides the vitamins and supplements, Stand Alone Fitness is also about exercising in your own environment and using the resources you have available to you. These resources could be store bought equipment or made in nature. As simple as a park bench to do step ups, knee lifts, and elevated pushups. Being creative and using your own body weight as resistance is a wonderful way to exercise.

Stand Alone Fitness is about becoming the healthiest you can be whether it involves your mind, body or soul. For me personally, it is truly a new identity and an amazing opportunity to share with others.

The future is what we make it and we should begin to shout it to the world from this day forward! We all have the ability to inspire others.

Come along and discover for yourself, the ways you can become the healthiest **You** in today's world.

As you continue to read, you will learn about the many ailments that we deal with on a regular basis. The ailments that get diagnosed and treated the most. While most doctors are quick to prescribe medications, why not consider alternatives?

Trust me, I do not have anything against doctors & nurses. Obviously if you read my story, you would know how much they did for me. I loved 99% of the nurses, doctors and surgeons I interacted with.

It's just that there is so much more out there to consider. Many natural alternatives that will help you with your ailment without the side effects that lead to more medications. In fact, these alternatives could actually save your life!

You owe it to yourself to know and learn a different way of healing yourself.

We will describe the ailment, mention what the most common treatment is and then give you the vitamin and/or mineral type that could be better for you.

Please do not be like me and just stop taking your prescribed medications without consulting your care provider first.

I simply decided it was in my best interest and I was in charge of what I put in my body. I made my own choice/decisions and I am content with that.

Note: As you look through this book, you may see the ailments listed are in alphabetic order. Please, by all means, jump around to the ailments that most interest you and pique' your curiosity to know more about.

Immune System

Let's start off by talking about your Immune System and what it does for you

According to the Cleveland Clinic, "your immune system is a large network of organs, white blood cells, proteins (antibodies) and chemicals. This system works together to protect you from foreign invaders (bacteria, viruses, parasites, and fungi) that cause infection, illness, and disease."

There are two parts of the immune system;

The innate immune system

This is your rapid response system. It is the first to take action when it finds an invader. It is made up of the skin, the eye's cornea, and the mucous membrane that lines the respiratory, gastrointestinal, and genitourinary tracts. These create physical barriers to help protect your body.

They protect against harmful germs, parasites, or even cells (such as cancer). The innate immune system is inherited. It is active from the moment you are born. When this system recognizes an invader, it goes to work right away.

The cells of this immune system surround and cover the invader. The invader is killed inside the immune system cells or also known as phagocytes.

The acquired immune system

The acquired immune system, with help from the innate system, makes special proteins called antibodies to protect your body from a specific invader. These antibodies are developed by cells called B lymphocytes after the body has been exposed to the invader.

The antibodies stay in your body. It can take several days for antibodies to form. Though after the first exposure, the immune system will recognize the invader and defend against it.

The acquired immune system changes during your life cycle. Immunizations train your immune system to make antibodies to protect them from harmful diseases such as Polio, Smallpox, and Mumps just to name a few.

The cells of both parts of the immune system are made in different organs of the body and are listed below;

- **Adenoids.** Two glands located at the back of the nasal passage.
- **Bone marrow.** The soft, spongy tissue found in bone cavities.
- **Lymph nodes.** Small organs shaped like beans, which are located all over the body and connect via the lymphatic vessels.
- **Lymphatic vessels.** A network of channels all over the body that carries lymphocytes to the lymphoid organs and bloodstream.
- **Peyer patches.** Lymphoid tissue in the small intestine.
- **Spleen.** A fist-sized organ located in the belly (abdominal) cavity.

- **Thymus.** Two lobes which join in front of the windpipe (trachea) behind the breastbone.
- **Tonsils.** Two oval masses in the back of the throat.

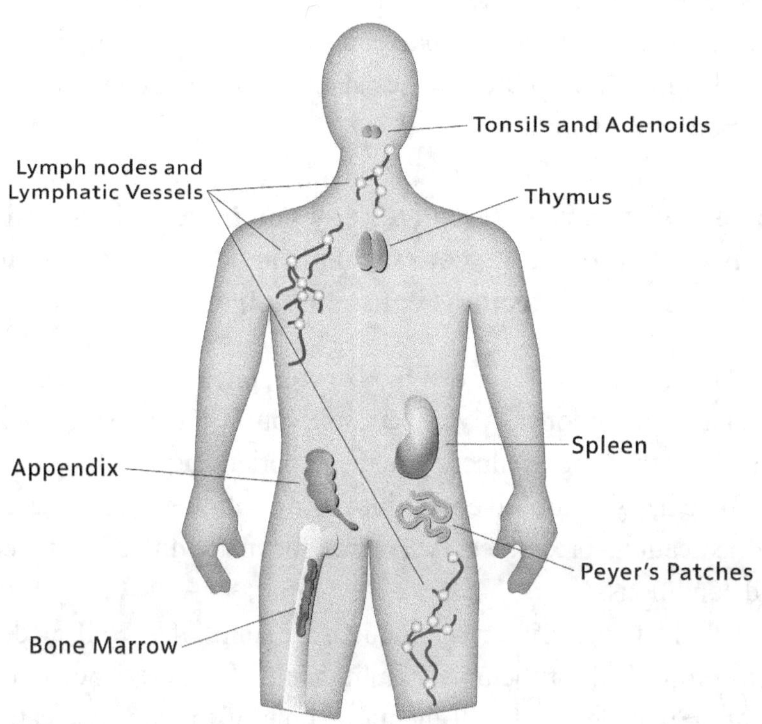

Your body needs antibiotics to help fight off infections and here is how this happens.

Antibiotics were developed and created to kill certain bacteria. Not all antibiotics are created equal. An antibiotic used for a skin ailment, probably isn't going to work on bacteria causing something like diarrhea. By using the wrong antibiotic or even too much can have an adverse effect in fact.

Antibiotic Resistance

While most colds and acute bronchitis infections won't respond to antibiotics and taking antibiotics too often or for the wrong reasons can change bacteria so much that antibiotics don't work against them. This is called bacterial resistance or antibiotic resistance. Some bacteria are now resistant to even the most powerful antibiotics available.

Have you ever heard a doctor say you have a virus and it just needs to run its course? This is because antibiotics don't work for infections caused by viruses.

Antibiotics are prescribed by a doctor, physician assistant and/or a nurse practitioner. Always consult your healthcare provider to determine the type of illness you are experiencing.

Whether you are given antibiotics or not, there are thousands of medications prescribed every year for many different ailments and conditions.

Our focus here is on alternatives to some, if not all medications prescribed for the most common ailments experienced in the United States today. I will mention some of the top medications used for each ailment but will focus on the alternative vitamins and minerals in supplement form that can be used instead, with great results.

So, let's get going!

ALLERGIES

As you know, your immune system produces proteins, known as antibodies to help protect the body from unwanted invaders. These invaders can make you sick and/or cause infections. In some people, the immune system produces antibodies against different substances that are eaten or inhaled which causes an allergic reaction. These are called allergens.

An allergen is a type of antigen that produces an abnormal immune response in which the immune system fights off a perceived threat that would otherwise be harmless to the body. Such reactions are called allergies.

The antibodies release several chemicals like histamines, that can cause irritation to sinuses, airways, skin and/or digestive system as a defense mechanism.

While I do not have allergies, I know so many people who do, including my youngest son and his mother. Their allergies consist of pollen, animal dander, mold and dust mites but there are plenty of other allergies. While I feel sorry for my son when he has a reaction but am kind of amazed when I hear him sneezing 14 times in a row. Yes, I have counted at times.

Different types of allergies

Food allergies; consist of things such as peanuts, shellfish, tree nuts, eggs, soy, fish, milk wheat, and tree nuts to name a few. What is even scarier is the fact, some don't even need to digest these foods. Simply being in proximity of them can cause life-threatening irritability.

Insect Bites/Stings; Being stung by a bee or wasps can create life-threatening challenges. Bites from other insects can cause rashes and other skin ailments. I know of this personally.

I was on a walk and almost home when I was bit or stung by something. Let me tell you, I jumped and it was very painful. In the coming days, a rash the size of a fist took over my calf.

It wasn't painful from the bite or sting anymore but it led to severe itchiness and the more I scratched it to relieve the annoyance, the bigger it got. Heck, I even drew blood on several occasions from all the scratching.

Eventually, I learned how to scratch it without the pain and/ or breaking the skin but yet, I got relief. I will explain more about what I did in the treatment segment of the ailment involved.

Latex; without getting into all these rather large fancy medical terms and names, most people who are allergic to latex are actually allergic to a protein found in the natural rubber tree from which latex is produced from.

When you are exposed to latex, your immune system starts to produce what is called IgE antibodies. It is the antibodies that cause the allergic reaction.

Healthcare workers and others who have to wear latex gloves for work are at a higher risk of developing a latex allergy. Also, people who have had a high number of surgeries can develop the allergy to latex as well as those who work in the rubber industry.

Medications; An abnormal reaction of the immune system to a medication is considered a drug allergy. Such drug allergies can be from prescribed medications, over the counter less strength medication and even some natural herbs can cause a reaction.

While most allergies to medication only cause minor skin rashes and hives, they may take a period of time to first be seen or felt. Others have experienced greater side-effects and a small percentage can be life-threatening.

One of the most common drug allergies is to Penicillin. As many as 10% of people report being allergic to this widely used class of antibiotic, making it the most commonly reported drug allergy.

A number of factors influence your chances of having a reaction to a medication including: body size, body chemistry, an underlying disease or even genetics.

Symptoms For Type of Allergy;

Hay Fever – Most outdoor plant allergens fall under this category.

- Runny Nose and Nasal Congestion
- Itchy Nose & Itchy Roof of Mouth/Throat
- Watery & Itchy Eyes
- Sneezing

Food Allergies –

- Tingly Mouth & Tongue
- Swelling of Lips, Tongue, Eyes & Throat
- Rashes & Hives
- Anaphylaxis

Insect Bite/Sting Allergies –

- Redness of Bite/Sting Site
- Itching on Site and/or Hives All Over Body
- Shortness of Breath, Tightness of Chest, Wheezing & Coughing
- Anaphylaxis

Latex Allergies –

- Reddening of Skin
- Itchy Skin
- Flaking/Peeling
- Discoloration

Drug Allergies –

- Rash Or Hives
- Itchy Skin
- Face Swelling
- Wheezing/Coughing
- Anaphylaxis

How are allergies diagnosed?

You are asked about symptoms you have experienced and other signs. You may be asked for a record of your dietary consumption over a period of time or there is a skin test and a blood test that can be performed.

The skin test consists of having different types of material, in small amounts, injected into the skin. This will cause hives (small bumps) at the test site if you are allergic.

The blood test or RAST Test (radioallergosorbent) measures your immune system's reaction and response time to specific allergens by measuring the amount of allergy-causing antibodies in the bloodstream.

Usual Treatment

- **Avoidance** – The most common treatment is avoidance. As crazy as it sounds, one should stay away from the things causing our body irritations once they are identified. If you have a peanut allergy, stay away from peanut butter sandwiches, peanut butter cups, peanut butter cookies!

Okay, I know I was being silly but these items, as delicious as they are, are truly killers to some people. This is the reality of it and a very scary one for those folks.

Would you know what to do if someone was having an allergic reaction to peanuts or another food related allergy? I know I wouldn't but perhaps I should find out! As should you because you may be surprised by the number in your inner circle who have these types of allergies. You could even save their life!

Other treatments include decongestants such as inhalers. When the pollen count gets extremely high, I know people who bring out their "puffers" as they call them. This allows them to open their airways to be able to breath.

I am thankful my son doesn't have or need a "puffer" but some day down the road, his allergies could worsen and he may need to have one on standby just in case.

- **Immunotherapy** – is another treatment involving allergy shots, generally given on a regular basis over a period of months to years. This is to decrease your sensitivity to the allergen. Another form of immunotherapy is a sublingual tablet that's placed under the tongue until it dissolves. Sublingual drugs are used to treat pollen allergies.

- **Epinephrine** – Also known as the EpiPen and/or Auvi-Q, are injectors that those who have experienced a severe allergy reaction, carry at all times. Their lives depend on an immediate injection of an epinephrine shot or they could and probably would die without it.

Of course, any type of medication carries its own side-effects. What if there were more natural ways to lessen the symptoms and dependance on medications? What would this look like?

Healthy Alternatives

- Vitamin C takes action as a natural antihistamine to help reduce the amount of histamine the body produces to protect the body from allergens. It also helps relieve symptom like runny nose, sneezing, watery eyes and congestion caused by allergens. Vitamin C also acts as a powerful antioxidant helping boost the immune system.
- Vitamin A & D have a powerful impact on immune cell's development and help suppress and prevent induction of autoimmune encephalomyelitis though more studies in humans are needed.
- Vitamin E is an antioxidant promoting health in blood, brain and skin. It also helps to decrease inflammation in the lungs and airways.
- Vitamin B6 has been shown to relieve bronchial constriction and even reduce the mucosal blockage of the airway as well as helping your body make proteins is essential to the immune system.
- Zinc is key to helping the body fight off viruses and bacteria

- Turmeric could possibly help minimize the swelling and irritation caused by allergic rhinitis and has the active ingredient curcumin, linked to reducing symptoms of several inflammation-driven diseases.

Please do not stop taking your prescribed medications like I did without consulting your care provider first.

ANXIETY

"**O**h my gosh, I am so overwhelmed! What am I going to do?" Anxiety affects us from time to time and it's okay and even healthy to get anxious now and then. It's when we are in a constant state of anxiety which can have serious health consequences.

We can experience anxiety in every day activities. Whether it is taking an exam or needing to do public speaking, trying to follow direction or even crossing a busy intersection.

When it becomes excessive, all-consuming, and begins to interfere with your daily life it is an indicator of underlying conditions.

I certainly know this to be true because I have dealt with anxiety off and on over the decades. Some self-induced as well as working several jobs where you needed to be alert and posing some anxiety.

I worked jobs operating heavy equipment on construction jobs and there were times if I wasn't alert and/or a bit anxious, I wouldn't be here to write this book. Examples of this were operating a quad dump truck and having to back up to the edge of a 200-foot cliff.

While dumping, the load could get hung up or the ground could give way or even have the box pull you over. It was enough anxiety to have my door open just in case I needed to jump.

Another instance was when I backed up to the excavator that was digging a hole to the left of my truck. After the first bucket was dumped in the box, I felt my truck shift and knew if I were to try and pull forward, the truck would plummet into the 25-foot-deep hole. You should have heard the chatter on the CB radio as everyone was alerted and a plan was put into action to save me and my boss' truck.

Anxiety can also cause you to do things you wouldn't ordinarily do. Like putting regular unleaded fuel in a truck which needed diesel fuel. Yes, I did this because I was anxious about something else going on in my life at the time.

There are several types of anxiety disorders and each come with their own characteristics and symptoms.

Anxiety Disorder – mental health disorder characterized by feelings of worry, anxiety, or fear strong enough to interfere with one's daily activities. Examples of this type of anxiety disorder include panic attacks, obsessive-compulsive disorder, and post-traumatic stress disorder.

Common Symptoms;

- Excessive Worry
- Paranoia
- Heart Palpitations

Generalized Anxiety Disorder (GAD) – Occurs at any age. Key component of GAD is continual and excessive worry about several different things you are dealing with in life. Like any anxiety disorder, someone with GAD can become paranoid with the status of money, health, family, work as well as other issues in their life. When this type of worry affects you, it begins to take over and consume your life in a negative manner.

Common Symptoms;

- Emotional Distress
- Fear
- Severe Anxiety

Social Anxiety Disorder – Everyday social interactions cause irrational anxiety, fear, self-consciousness, and embarrassment for people suffering from social anxiety disorder. The idea of being judged, embarrassed or humiliated, and/or concern of offending others is a mental health condition that keeps people from living a full life.

Common Symptoms;

- Depression
- Palpitations
- Fear

Obsessive Compulsive Disorder – is a common and chronic disorder in which a person has uncontrollable, reoccurring obsessions and/or compulsive behaviors which they feel the urge to repeat over and over. This disorder can develop over time and can turn into dangerous coping mechanisms such as doing dangerous activities, having a fear of germs and/or even needing to arrange things in a particular order in order to feel safe.

Common Symptoms;

- Fear of contamination
- Doubts and needing things orderly
- Difficult tolerating uncertainty

Separation Anxiety – Most of the time, this disorder affects children who become separated from parents and become excessively anxious. This disorder can affect children well into adulthood but then taper off over time.

Common Symptoms;

- Fear of losing family/friends
- Self-doubt
- Blaming self for others leaving

This disorder hits close to home for me as I was adopted 3 times and in 4 homes before I was 5 ½ years old.

Even after I was adopted for the last time, my separation anxiety was reinforced on a camping trip. When we arrived, I hit it off with the older girl in the campsite next to ours, only to wake up the next morning and they were gone. I stood in the middle of our tent crying. What did I do to cause this?

It happened a few years later when my family went to the Black Hills for a week and there was an older teenage girl who took a liking to me. She took me horseback riding several times and played the guitar. One morning, she was gone. I was crushed.

Again, what did I do to make people come into my life, only to leave me again? Side note, my relationships in high school were very superficial as I was too worried I would get attached to someone. In fact, when I dated, I would break it off before the other person could do it.

This made me feel like I was in control of my feelings and not getting hurt again. Yes, I lost out on some special relationships because of this.

I am sure, this is why I still have trust issues when it comes to relationships.

Overall Causes of Anxiety (Included but are not limited to)

- change in living arrangements
- stress at work or home
- complications in relationships
- emotional shock following a stressful or traumatic event
- verbal, sexual, physical or emotional abuse or trauma
- death or loss of a loved one

Usual Treatment

- **Psychotherapy** (therapy/counseling) When it comes to psychotherapy, there are an array of treatments and services to explore, depending on severity. Some people may need simple relaxation techniques while others may need other corrective measures to help them cope and/or overcome their anxiety disorder.

    Other therapies include corrective breathing exercises, building self-esteem, cognitive therapy, learning to be assertive, structural problem solving, and being mindful of what causes one to worry and overly stress out.

- **Medications** – Prozac is probably the most well-known medication prescribed for those suffering from one anxiety or another but there is also Zoloft, Paxil, Lexapro, and even Celexa to name another. Each one comes with pros and cons. The question comes down to what side-effects one can live with when deciding to use a drug to help ease the level of discomfort associated with the anxiety being treated.

    I once had a friend who was on three different medications for her anxiety symptoms. One medication to ease the anxiety, another medication to help with a side-effect and another medication to help with a side-effect of the secondary medication. At one point, the friend became self-harming because the increased anxiety they were enduring.

It wasn't until it was suggested she get off all the medications to see where she was at mentally, that this person was able to grasp their reality and make necessary changes.

I am not a big advocate of medications much less for anxieties that can be lessened and/or overcome with other natural remedies.

Healthy Alternatives

- Research shows certain vitamins and minerals help to reduce anxiety symptoms. They include; **magnesium, vitamin D, saffron, omega-3s, chamomile, L-theanine, vitamin C, and curcumin.**
- **Magnesium** – binds to calming receptors in the body to block more stimulating neurotransmitters' activity, results in a more restful state. It helps to regulate the release of stress hormones like cortisol. Helps your nervous system.
- **Vitamin D** – decreases anxiety levels significantly, especially in women suffering from type 2 diabetes. Some studies suggest a common link between the vitamin D deficiency and anxiety disorders.
- **Saffron** – is a compound that reduces anxiety and increases one's mood.
- **Omega-3s** might help ease anxiety symptoms in people diagnosed with a range of physical and mental health problems.
- **Chamomile** – is a popular natural remedy and may be effective in decreasing anxiety disorders. It has been shown to cause anxiety relief as a relaxation component.

- **L-theanine** – has an anti-anxiety effect by helping to increase levels of dopamine and serotonin in the brain, resulting in the feeling of calmness.
- **Vitamin C** – works to clear the body of excess cortisol produced during times of stress and turmoil. Lowering cortisol in the system often helps to reduce the feeling of stress and anxiety. Vitamin C also helps blood sugar levels from raising during stressful circumstances.
- **Curcumin** – helps boost dopamine and serotonin levels which in return, help treat anxiety and depression.

Please do not stop taking your prescribed medications like I did without consulting your care provider first.

ARTHRITIS

Inflammation of the joints, causing pain, stiffness, and in some cases, deformities. While there are more than 100 types of arthritis, there are two types which are most commonly diagnosed and treated. They are Osteoarthritis and Rheumatoid arthritis.

Osteoarthritis (OA) – is the wearing down of the protective tissue at the ends of bones called cartilage which occurs gradually and worsens over time. This commonly causes pain in the hands, neck, lower back, knees and hips.

Rheumatoid arthritis (RA) – is a chronic inflammatory disorder affecting many joints, including those in the hands and feet. Here the body's immune system attacks its own tissue, including joints. In severe cases, it attacks internal organs. It also affects joint linings, causing painful swelling. Over time, rheumatoid arthritis can cause bone erosion and joint deformities.

Growing up, I remember cracking my knuckles and other things such as my neck and back. When I cracked my knuckles, I was told my knuckles would get 3 times the size of my fingers.

When I cracked my neck, I was told that one day, I would crack my neck and become stuck in one position, have my head tilted to one side or become paralyzed.

40 years later, I still crack my knuckles and neck to relieve pressure. Unfortunately, I have too much mid-section girth to be able to crack the back. Of course, when I see the way my son cracks his back, I am both jealous and concerned about what his body will be like when he gets to be my age. I guess he should enjoy it while he can.

I do know a lot of people who are suffering from either one of these two types of arthritis, especially women. I was actually shocked to learn women are 3 times more likely to experience and deal with arthritis.

Causes/Risk Factors

- Wear and tear of a joint from overuse. Take professional basketball players for instance. They put a lot of stress on their ankle, knee and hip joints even though the floor they play on has some give to it. After a 10-year career, see how many of them walk and move around now. Their bodies, especially their joints have taken such a beating!
- Age, OA is most common in adults over age 50. If you are over 25 years old, you have most likely heard a parent or grandparent complain about their aches and pains. Most of this is from their arthritis.
- Injuries, one of the most common causes of arthritis. When an injury occurs in a joint and doesn't heal properly, it can cause arthritis to form as well as cause the cartilage to deteriorate over time. This leads to pain and stiffness as well as bone on bone scraping which is extremely painful.
- Obesity is another common cause of either OA or RA, especially in the U.S. where there is an overweight problem. I can say this as I too am overweight. Think about it this way, carrying an extra 40 pounds will stress out your knees, hips, and ankles by 160 pounds of pressure with every step.

For those who are only 10 pounds overweight, you are still adding 40 pounds of added pressure to your hips, knees and ankles. This is insane! No wonder we are starting to see more and more people in wheelchairs at a younger age.

- Autoimmune disorders (RA) can affect the condition of your joints and cause arthritis. Autoimmune disorders mistake good cells for bad and will attack the normal cells, causing your immune system to attack the lining of your joints.

- Genetics are another cause of arthritis. Come on, you knew this was going to be mentioned. You can now blame your mom, dad, grandpa, grandma and beyond for your body make up. As mentioned earlier, your body's weight can have an effect on whether you some day develop arthritis and your genes could contribute to it.

- Muscle weakness is a factor and/or perhaps a byproduct of joint damage and arthritis.

Usual Treatment

- **Low-Impact Exercises** – low-impact aerobic exercises are easier on your joints include walking, bicycling, swimming and using an elliptical machine.

- **Nonsteroidal anti-inflammatory drugs (NSAIDs)** can relieve pain and reduce inflammation. Examples include ibuprofen (Advil, Motrin IB, others) and naproxen sodium (Aleve).

- **Biologic Medications** – Such as Humira, Enbrel, Orencia, Rituxan, and Remicade

Healthy Alternatives

- **Curcumin** (from turmeric root) Evidence suggests the turmeric root has anti-inflammatory properties.
- **Vitamin D** has an anti-inflammatory effect on the health of bones and is essential to help prevent the thinning of the bones and works against the inflammation of arthritis.
- **Omega-3 Fatty Acids** are thought to have immunomodulatory properties as they act as precursors to lipid mediators of inflammation which may limit or modulate the inflammatory response.
- **Glucosamine and Chondroitin Sulfate** protect cells called chondrocytes, which help maintain cartilage structure, the potential to slow cartilage deterioration in the joints, and to reduce pain in the process.

CANCER (IN GENERAL)

Abnormal cells which divide uncontrollably and have the ability to infiltrate and destroy normal body tissue. These abnormal cells can develop anywhere in the body and also spread throughout the body very quickly. There are cancers that form tumors while other forms of cancer do not.

A cancer can continue to grow and push onto organs, nerves, and blood vessels. The pressure created in some forms of cancer cause some of the signs and symptoms of the particular cancer. Fatigue, fever, and/or unexplained weight loss can be symptoms of cancer.

Cancerous cells use up much of the body's source of energy.

While there are many forms of cancer, listed are the most common types;

- **Breast Cancer** – A cancer which forms in the cells of the breasts.
- **Prostate Cancer** – A cancer in a man's prostate, a small walnut-sized gland that produces seminal fluid.
- **Basal Cell Cancer** – A type of skin cancer which begins in the basal cells.

- **Melanoma** – The most serious type of skin cancer.
- **Colon Cancer** – A cancer of the colon or rectum, located at the digestive tract's lower end.
- **Lung Cancer** – A cancer that begins in the lungs and most often occurs in people who smoke.
- **Leukemia** – A cancer of blood-forming tissues, hindering the body's ability to fight infection.
- **Lymphoma** – A cancer of the lymphatic system.

Causes/Risk Factors

- A gene mutation may instruct a healthy cell to grow too fast and divided, creating a mass of new abnormal cells.
- Some gene mutations are inherited but most occur after you're born.
- Because cancer can take decades to develop, it's most common in people aged 65 and older. However, it can occur at any age.
- Certain lifestyle choices are known to increase your risk of cancer. Such as smoking, excessive alcohol use, excessive exposure to the sun, being overweight, and lack of exercise.
- Harmful chemicals in the environment can increase your risk of cancer. Examples include secondhand smoke, asbestos and benzene.
- Over consumption of processed meats, alcohol, and tobacco products.
- Obesity puts a real strain on your immune system.
- Exposure to radiation, including ultraviolet radiation from the sun.

Usual Treatment

The big 3 for treatment of cancer is surgery, chemotherapy, and radiation.

1. **Surgery** – Surgery is a procedure in which a surgeon removes cancer from your body. It works best for solid tumors that are contained in one area. Of course, there are other types of surgeries and procedures performed for the removal of cancer cells. They are lasers, cryosurgery, hyperthermia, and photodynamic therapy.
2. **Chemotherapy** – A drug treatment using powerful drugs to kill cancerous cells in the body. The drug combination usually consists of cisplatin, melphalan, busulfan, cyclophosphamide, capecitabine, and 5-fluorouracil just to name a few.
3. **Radiation** – Known as radiation therapy (radiotherapy), is a cancer treatment which uses high doses of radiation to kill cancer cells and shrink cancerous tumors. Mainly used in the beginning but also after surgery.

Other Treatments;

- Hormone Therapy is a treatment which slows or stops the growth of breast and prostate cancers that use hormones to grow.
- Immunotherapy is a type of cancer treatment that helps your immune system fight cancer.
- Photodynamic Therapy uses a drug activated by light to kill cancer and other abnormal cells.
- Hyperthermia is a type of treatment in which body tissue is heated to as high as 113 °F to help damage and kill cancer cells with little or no harm to normal tissue.

Healthy Alternatives

- **Vitamin D** has been found to have several active properties which slow or prevent the development of cancer, including promoting cellular differentiation, decreasing cancer cell growth, stimulating cell death (apoptosis), and reducing tumor blood vessel formation according to studies of cancer cells and of tumors in mice.
- **Vitamin A** intake may contribute to a lower risk of developing a common form of skin cancer.
- **Vitamin C** this antioxidant may forage reactive oxygen strain preventing DNA damage and other effects important in cancer transformation.
- **Vitamin E** has been shown to inhibit tumor formation due to its antioxidant components. Some studies suggest vitamin E may contribute to reducing the risk of prostate cancer.
- **Turmeric** reduces inflammation, which is at the root of many diseases, including cancer. It has the potential to prevent and treat cancer. Animal and lab studies show turmeric can help prevent cancer growth and kill certain cancer cells, but more studies are needed in humans.
- **Omega-3 Fish Oil** has been suggested by experts to help protect against cancer. Omega-3 fatty acids also helps to reduce inflammation in the body. This is good news considering the fact several cancers are linked to inflammation. Omega-3 Fish Oil may improve the overall survival of cancer patients.

CHRONIC FATIGUE SYNDROME (CFS)

A medical condition of unknown cause, with fever, aching, and prolonged tiredness and depression, typically occurring after a viral infection. Characterized by profound fatigue, sleep abnormalities, pain, and other symptoms which are made worse by exertion. While there is no known cause, chronic fatigue syndrome occurs more times in women and may include environmental or genetic factors.

More than not, the main symptom is fatigue, over a long period of time even though resting doesn't help. There is no known cure nor is there an approved treatment for this ailment. Some symptoms are treated like other ailments to help lessen the discomfort and provide relief of other symptoms.

There is no single test to confirm a diagnosis of chronic fatigue syndrome.

Causes/Risk Factors

- While there is no known singular cause for this ailment, some experts believe chronic fatigue syndrome is connected to viral infection and/or psychological stress.

- CFS isn't even diagnosed until after a period of 6 months of symptoms that can become so severe, it interferes with your normal daily activities, both at home and at work.
- Rest and sleep don't seem to help.
- CFS can worsen as we age, making it more difficult to perform already difficult tasks.
- CFS is an ailment even the best diet or exercise routine can not help control.
- Mental health issues, family health history, past infections such as colds, flu, or stomach bug can activate and/or worsen symptoms of CFS.

Usual Treatment

As mentioned, there is no known cure or approved treatment for this ailment. Most of the symptoms are treated separately in the following ways;

- **Self-Care** Management of one's stresses and learning relaxation techniques including yoga, medication, and hypnosis.
- **Medications** usually antidepressants are prescribed to help with one's anxiety and coping.
- **Support Groups** that have counselors as well as others who have suffered from CFS to help share experiences with people who suffer with similar conditions.

Healthy Alternatives

- **Vitamin E** helps to relieve pain in CFS sufferers. It can also improve leg cramps at night, which interfere with sleep.

- **Vitamin B12** helps increase energy and studies suggest that low levels of B12 may contribute to chronic fatigue syndrome as well as fibromyalgia.
- **Vitamin D3** has shown to improve muscle mitochondrial cell function, correlated with an improvement in symptoms of myopathy and fatigue.
- **Selenium** Supports immune function by enhancing antibody production.
- **Magnesium** is a natural muscle pain reliever and helps the body increase its production of DHEA, a hormone with favorable effects on memory, stress, sleep and depression.
- **Calcium** is needed in every cell of the body and is key in helping the immune system demolish a virus or infection.
- **CoQ10** helps to replenish the abnormal levels of CoQ10 in plasma and muscle tissue. Some healthcare providers recommended as much as 200 mg per day for CFS.

Please do not stop taking your prescribed medications like I did without consulting your care provider first.

Coronary Artery Disease (CAD)

When I think of coronary artery disease, there are many heart related issues that come to mind. Whether it might be a heart attack, chest pain, dizziness, nausea, sleep disturbances, cold sweats, neck pain, and/or weakness, it is wise to get it checked out before it is too late.

Causes/risk factors

The biggest culprit is cholesterol, a waxy substance that sticks to the inner lining of the artery wall, forming what is known as plaque. Over time, the plaque begins to block the artery, causing some of the symptoms listed above until either its discovered or it causes a major health crisis.

Again, symptoms can be different from person to person but if you have blood flow to the heart become blocked, this can result in a heart attack. When the heart suddenly stops pumping blood through the heart to the rest of the body, this is known as cardiac arrest.

- **High Blood Pressure** also known as hypertension is a disease that develops when blood flows through arteries at higher-than-normal pressure. blood pressure is made up of two numbers: systolic and diastolic. Systolic pressure is the pressure when the ventricles pump blood out of the heart. Diastolic pressure is the pressure between heartbeats when the heart is filling with blood. 120/80 is normal. 130/80 is considered high blood pressure.

- **Age** causes arteries to stiffen, called arteriosclerosis or hardening of the arteries. This is normal with growing older.
- **Environment** is another factor as working around toxins can put you at greater risk. Having a lot of stress at work, sitting for long periods of time, and interrupted sleep patterns place greater stress on your body.
- **Genetics** is something you can't take for granted. Finding out your family health history can go a long way to avoiding trouble and even preventing **CAD** further down the road.
- **Physical Inactivity** can worsen other heart related risk factors such as high blood pressure, high blood cholesterol, obesity, and diabetes.
- **Smoking** or even second-hand smoke can lead to health issues which puts a lot of stress on your heart.
- **Diet & Lifestyle** have a huge impact on your health and can be the difference between a healthy life or of heart related chronic illnesses.
- **Race & Ethnicity** plays a big part in the people who experience coronary heart disease. CAD is the leading cause of death for people of most racial and ethnic groups in the United States, including African Americans. For Hispanics, Asian Americans or Pacific Islanders, and American Indians or Alaska Natives, heart disease is second only to cancer.
- **Gender** also plays a role as to when one can expect to deal with heart related issues. Coronary heart disease affects men and women while obstructive coronary artery disease is more common in men. Non-obstructive coronary disease

is more common in women. In men, the risk for coronary heart disease starts to increase around age 45 while women have a lower risk of coronary heart disease until around the age of 55.

Usual Treatment

Your treatment for coronary artery disease depends on how serious your condition and/or symptoms are. Several tests are given to determine the severity of the problem. Those tests are as follows;

- **Stress Test** used to judge your activity level. You are asked to walk/run on a treadmill. There are usually four stages, each one more difficult than the latter. During this test, the technician is monitoring your progress and looking for irregularities in your heart rhythm. The results are usually passed onto a cardiologist to review if immediate care isn't needed. 60% accurate.
- **Nuclear Stress Test** uses a small amount of radioactive material (tracer) and an imaging machine to create pictures showing the blood flow to your heart. 70% accurate.
- **Calcium-score Screening Heart Scan**, also known as a Heart CT (computerized tomography) scan, is used to find calcium deposits in plaque buildup in the arteries of the heart.
- **Cardiac Catheterization** is used to diagnose and treat problems with your heart or blood vessels. A doctor specializing in this procedure, inserts a small tube called a catheter through your blood vessels and into your heart. This procedure is used to measure blockages of the arteries and to determine if a stent can be placed to help open up the artery to increase blood flow. It is also used to check the

heart's valves, take samples of your heart tissue (biopsy) among other issues.

Diet and Exercise are crucial to maintain a healthy heart and live a long life. While CAD is not necessarily a death sentence, keeping a healthy diet and exercising regularly can keep the heart strong and also keep the arteries of the heart from clogging.

Managing Stress is another way to help prolong your life and prevent a dangerous heart health event. Learning how to cope with problems, learning how to relax through meditation and yoga, and improving your overall emotional health.

Stop Smoking will take stress off not only your lungs but your heart as well. There is scientific evidence showing nicotine damages your heart so just **STOP!**

Quality Sleep is important to maintaining a healthy lifestyle. Most experts suggest getting between 7-9 hours of sleep daily for good health. This also helps relieve stress on the heart as well as the body as a whole.

Medications are prescribed pretty regular, whether it's to lower blood pressure, lower cholesterol or to maintain a normal heart rhythm, these medications can have side-effects which can create other health issues. Here are what some of the most prescribed types of medications do;

- **ACE inhibitors and beta blockers** help lower blood pressure and decrease how hard your heart is working.
- **Calcium channel blockers** lower blood pressure by allowing blood vessels to relax.
- **Medicines to control blood sugar,** such as empagliflozin, canagliflozin, and liraglutide, can help lower your risk

for complications if you have coronary heart disease and diabetes.

- **Metformin** controls plaque buildup if you have diabetes.
- **Nitrates,** such as nitroglycerin, dilate your coronary arteries and relieve or prevent chest pain from angina.
- **Ranolazine** treats coronary microvascular disease and the chest pain it may cause.
- **Statins or non-statin therapies** control high blood cholesterol. You may need statin therapy if you have a higher risk of coronary heart disease or stroke or if you have diabetes and are between ages 40 and 75.

Healthy Alternatives

- **CoQ10** helps to replenish the abnormal levels of CoQ10 in plasma and muscle tissue. Studies have shown CoQ10 can increase HDL-C and ApoA1 levels and might help reduce the chance for CAD. CoQ10 also helps lower the levels of inflammatory biomarkers shown to be risk factors associated with coronary artery disease.
- **Vitamin C (ascorbic acid)** is seen as an anti-oxidant. Some people feel vitamin C is a good treatment for heart disease. Some studies have shown vitamin C supplements lower blood pressure but taking too much of it can potentially cause hardening of the arteries. It is encouraged to not exceed the daily recommended dose.
- **Vitamin E** has been associated with lower risk of coronary heart disease in middle-aged to older men and women. Some research studies suggest vitamin E as an antioxidant can reduce cardiovascular disease by trapping free radicals.
- **Vitamin B12** and folic acid may help prevent heart disease by lowering the body's levels of homocysteine according to studies performed. Vitamin B12 is a nutrient which helps

keep your body›s blood and nerve cells healthy. It also helps make DNA, the genetic material in all of your cells. It is also known vitamin B12 helps prevent megaloblastic anemia, a blood condition that makes people tired and weak.

- **Resveratrol** thins the blood and keeps blood pressure in check. It might slow blood clotting as well. Resveratrol helps reduce low-density lipoprotein (LDL) cholesterol (the "bad" cholesterol) and potentially helps prevent damage to blood vessels.

Please do not stop taking your prescribed medications like I did without consulting your care provider first.

Depression

Put on a happy face and trudge on through it, right? Nope, not that easy but yet, many do this. In fact, most people suffering from depression won't really tell you how they are feeling or what they are enduring for several reasons. Mostly, embarrassment. We will get back to this in a moment but first, what is depression?

Depression is a disorder which negatively impacts your mood and your sense of self-worth. It is a serious ailment that has several sub-categories such as;

- **Bipolar Disorder** – a disorder in the brain which causes dramatic changes in one's mood, energy, and ability to perform daily activities. Bipolar disorder can last for days at a time without proper diagnosis and treatment.
- **Bipolar 2 Disorder** – a variant of a lessor degree of the mania episodes of bipolar 1 disorder. Also called hypomanic episode, which last as long as 4 days to 2 weeks at a time with extra energy, both happy and potentially irritable.
- **Clinical Depression** – also known as Major Depressive Disorder (MDD) or unipolar, clinical depression is described as major depression where one loses interest in activities, is sad and it lasts for long periods of time, usually longer than two weeks.

- **Persistent Depressive Disorder (PDD) – (formally dysthymic disorder)** is considered a mild but long-term form of depression involving both mental as well as behavioral disorders and is considered chronic depression.
- **Postpartum Depression** – occurs after child birth and causes difficulty bonding with child, insomnia, intense irritability, and loss of appetite.

Causes/Risk Factors

While there is one direct cause of depression, there are many factors which can lead to depression. These are;

- **Serious Illness** – Depression can develop due to a serious illness or even provoked by other medical conditions.
- **Abuse** – Emotional, physical, and sexual abuse provide the underlying condition or event for depression after the fact. This can last for years is not properly treated.
- **Major Changing Events** – Change can be overwhelming with even good events. Whether its graduating from school, starting a new career and/or simply starting a new chapter in one's life can have the ingredients for developing depression.
- **Age** – We change as we get older and with these changes, create the chances of developing depression. It is known that people who are older such as the elderly, are at a higher risk of depression. Whether it is living alone, or having a lacking support system, loneliness is a form or depression.
- **Medications** – A good portion of the medications prescribed today have a side-effect which increase the risk of depression.
- **Gender** – While depression can affect just about anyone, women are twice as likely to become depressed compared

to men. It is believed hormonal changes that women experience through their lives may play a factor.

- **Genes** – Do you have a family history of depression? If you know of this history, chances are, you will be more apt to one day be diagnosed with depression yourself as the risk factor increase greatly.
- **Conflict** – Personal conflicts with family and/or co-workers can lead to depression. As mentioned with genes, one can become more vulnerable to conflicts in one's life.
- **Other Personal Problems** – There is a wide variety of ways one can become depressed through social isolation, feelings of unworthiness, and fear of socializing in itself.
- **Death or Loss** – Sadness is a stage of grief which can lead to depression if left unchecked. Losing a loved one and/or perhaps losing a relationship can cause a downward spiral as you question the reasons for either. While sadness and grief are natural after a loss, prolonged periods of either puts you at greater risk of being diagnosed with some type of depression.
- **Substance Abuse** – it is known that approximately 30% of people who suffer from substance abuse issues may develop major or clinical depression in their lifetime.

Usual Treatments

Unfortunately, treatment for depression usually involves medications. Now I am not saying this is a bad thing altogether, but I do have experience working with someone who was taking medication for depression. Of course, they had a side-effect from prescribed medication which led to another prescribed medication and again, this led to another side-effect and another medication was prescribed.

This is called, "treating the symptom/side-effect" rather than treating the actual disease. The person I was working with was all over the board and had serious mood swings, especially when alcohol was involved. Eventually she decided to get off all prescribed medications and her life changed for the better.

Some of the medications prescribed are;

- **Selective serotonin reuptake inhibitors (SSRIs)** Typically the first line of treatment because they cause less side-effects and are deemed safer than other antidepressants. Some SSRIs include Prozac (fluoxetine), Paxil (paroxetine), Zoloft (sertraline), Celexa (citalopram), and Lexapro (escitalopram).
- **Serotonin and norepinephrine reuptake inhibitors (SNRIs)** These consist of Cymbalta (duloxetine), Effexor XR (venlafaxine), and Pristiq (desvenlafaxine).
- **Norepinephrine and dopamine reuptake inhibitors (NDRIs)** Many antidepressant medications can cause sexual side-effects. Anything from erectile dysfunction in men to low libido and vaginal dryness in women. Wellbutrin (bupropion) is one of the few antidepressants not frequently associated with sexual side effects.
- **Atypical antidepressants** According to Mayo Clinic, sedating drugs such as Remeron (trazodone & mirtazapine) don't fit very well into other antidepressant categories. Yet, Viibryd (Vilazodone has been known to have less of a sexual side-effect.
- **Tricyclic antidepressants** are considered some of the older types of antidepressants and have more severe side-effects compared to the newer antidepressants.
- **Monoamine oxidase inhibitors (MAOIs)** are prescribed when other antidepressants don't work. Some of the newer

developed drugs can be administered through the use of a skin patch, causing less side-effects.

Other forms of treatment;

- **Psychotherapy** is when the patient communicates with a mental health provider and talks about the symptoms, underlying conditions and other related issues. This helps to identify factors which contribute to the patient's depression which then can be used to help lessen and/or dissolve future bouts of depression. These sessions help to defuse situations and crises before they become difficult for the patient. One way it replaces negative thoughts with positive ones.
- **Electroconvulsive therapy (ECT)** is a procedure where electrical currents are passed through the brain. This therapy is used on patients who haven't had any relief from the usual medications tried and it is said ECT is thought to improve depression by effecting the levels of brain neurotransmitters. ECT is also used for patients who are unable to take medications due to a high risk of suicide or other health conditions.
- **Transcranial magnetic stimulation (TMS)** is a procedure where you sit in a reclining chair with a coil placed against your scalp. The coil sends brief magnetic pulses to stimulate nerve cells in your brain that are involved in mood regulation.

Healthy Alternatives

- **Vitamin D** is a fat-soluble vitamin and is often considered low in people with depression as well as other mental health disorders. Research has shown people over 65 with depression were 14% lower in vitamin D than healthy individuals. And while sunlight accounts for about 90% of the vitamin D daily intake for most people, supplementing might be needed. While Vitamin D is a key nutrient for your mood and mental health, be aware too much vitamin D can be toxic.

- **B12** is a water-soluble vitamin required for a healthy central nervous system, red blood cell formation, and DNA synthesis. A deficiency in B12 has been linked to psychiatric symptoms, such as: irritability, personality change, depression, dementia, and psychosis. B12 helps in the role of producing chemicals in the brain that affect mood and other brain function.

- **Niacin (B3)** is a water-soluble B vitamin critical for many functions in the brain, including mood. Although the average adult needs only about 14 to 16 mg of niacin daily, much higher doses have been shown to help some people with psychiatric disorders. Niacin is part of the metabolizing process of forming serotonin from tryptophan, an amino acid.

- **Folate (B9)** may help reduce depressive symptoms. Folate, a naturally occurring B vitamin, is needed in the brain for the synthesis of norepinephrine, serotonin, and dopamine.

- **Vitamin C**, or L-ascorbic acid, is a critical vitamin for several functions in the body, including immune function and the production of collagen and neurotransmitters. It also helps reduce chronic inflammation and oxidative stress, which research has shown may play a role in depression. Vitamin C has the ability to improve the body's normal response to stress. anti—oxidants in Vitamin-C play a therapeutic role and aid in coping with anxiety, stress, fatigue and mood swings.

- **Magnesium** blocks the activity of stimulating neurotransmitters and cohere to calming receptors, resulting in a more peaceful, resting state. It helps to regulate the release of stress hormones like cortisol, acting like the brake on your body's nervous system.
- **Zinc** has been shown to improve mood and lessen symptoms of depression. Zinc stabilizes cortisol levels over time.

Please do not stop taking your prescribed medications like I did without consulting your care provider first.

DIABETES

Diabetes is a disease that occurs when your blood glucose, also called blood sugar, is too high. Blood glucose is your main source of energy and comes from the food you eat. Insulin, a hormone made by the pancreas, helps glucose from food get into your cells to be used for energy.

While there is no known cure for diabetes at this time, you can lower your risk by changing your diet intake and exercising regularly as well as maintaining a healthy weight.

There are several types of diabetes and they are;

- **Type 2 diabetes** is a chronic condition which affects the way the body processes blood sugar (glucose). When a person is diagnosed with type 2 diabetes, it means the body doesn't produce enough insulin or it resists insulin. A person with this condition can experience hunger, fatigue, increased thirst, frequent urination, and even blurred vision.

- **Type 1 diabetes** also known as juvenile diabetes is chronic condition where the pancreas produces little to no insulin. Like type 2 diabetes, a person with this condition can experience hunger, fatigue, increased thirst, frequent urination, and even blurred vision.

- **Prediabetes** is a condition in which blood sugar is high, but not high enough to be type 2 diabetes. Has no symptoms and can be reversed with lifestyle changes, weight loss, and medications, and it is possible to bring a blood sugar level back to normal.

- **Gestational diabetes** is a type of diabetes which can develop during pregnancy in women who don't already have diabetes. While there are no symptoms with gestational diabetes, a blood test is conducted during the pregnancy to determine diagnosis.

Myself, I went from prediabetic to type 2 in a matter of months. Why? Because someone thought it was a good idea to change the blood sugar ranges. Yes, I said it! I was at a 6.3 and no where near 7.4 until the numbers got changed to 6.1. Maybe it was in order to promote more pharmaceuticals. Just my opinion but since I am writing this book, I am choosing to share my thoughts and opinion.

Causes/Risk Factors

A lot of people believe you have to be overweight/obese to develop diabetes and nothing could be further from the truth. As we have discovered, diabetes begins when your body doesn't produce enough insulin or the cells resist it.

Other factors besides the thought of fatty tissue are as follows but not limited to;

- **Inactivity** – You are at a greater risk the less active you are.
- **Race/ethnicity** – While it is unclear why, certain ethnicity groups are at great risks, including Black, American Indian, Hispanic, and Asian American people.
- **Family history** – If a parent or sibling has been diagnosed for diabetes, you are at a higher risk.

- **Age** – As we age, our risk of having to deal with the risks of diabetes also goes up. Loss of muscle, weight gain and exercising less seem to be the factors.
- **High blood pressure** – Having high blood pressure is a factor to greater the risk of diabetes.
- **Polycystic ovary syndrome** – Like women who can develop gestational diabetes during pregnancy, women with irregular menstrual periods are at greater risk.
- **High cholesterol & triglyceride levels** – having high numbers with bad cholesterol puts you at a greater risk of diabetes.

Because diabetes affects people differently, I want to share with you another category.

Complications

While long term complications of diabetes develop gradually, the longer you have it, the less control you have to fight it. Diabetes complications can become disabling and even be life-threatening. Complications include;

- **Cardiovascular disease.** Diabetes dramatically increases the risk of various cardiovascular problems, including coronary artery disease with chest pain (angina), heart attack, stroke and narrowing of arteries (atherosclerosis). If you have diabetes, you're more likely to have heart disease or a stroke.
- **Kidney damage (nephropathy).** The kidneys contain millions of tiny blood vessel clusters (glomeruli) that filter waste from your blood. Diabetes can damage this delicate filtering system. Severe damage can lead to kidney failure

or irreversible end-stage kidney disease, which may require dialysis or a kidney transplant.

- **Foot damage.** Nerve damage in the feet or poor blood flow to the feet increases the risk of various foot complications. Left untreated, cuts and blisters can develop serious infections, which often heal poorly. This can lead to becoming septic which is life-threatening. These infections may also require toe, foot or leg amputation.
- **Eye damage (retinopathy).** Diabetes can damage the blood vessels of the retina (diabetic retinopathy), potentially leading to blindness. Diabetes also increases the risk of other serious vision conditions, such as cataracts and glaucoma. Diabetes also contributes to blurred vision.
- **Nerve damage (neuropathy).** Excess sugar can injure the walls of the tiny blood vessels (capillaries) that nourish your nerves, especially in your legs. This can cause tingling, numbness, burning or pain which usually begins at the tips of the toes or fingers and gradually spreads upward. When left untreated, you could lose all sense of feeling in the affected limbs. Damage to the nerves related to digestion can cause problems with nausea, vomiting, diarrhea or constipation. For men, it could also lead to erectile dysfunction.
- **Skin conditions.** Diabetes may leave you more susceptible to skin problems, including bacterial and fungal infections.
- **Depression.** Depression symptoms are common in people with type 1 and type 2 diabetes. Depression can affect diabetes management.
- **Hearing impairment.** Hearing problems are more common in people with diabetes.
- **Alzheimer's disease.** Type 2 diabetes may increase the risk of dementia, such as Alzheimer's disease. The poorer your blood sugar control, the greater the risk appears to be.

Although there are theories as to how these disorders might be connected, none has yet been proved.

Usual Treatments

Most diabetes treatment starts with tests to determine what type of diabetes you are dealing with. These tests include;

- **Hemoglobin (A1C) test.** This blood test indicates your average blood sugar level for the past two to three months. It does this by measuring the percentage of blood sugar attached to hemoglobin, the oxygen-carrying protein in red blood cells. The higher your blood sugar levels, the more hemoglobin you'll have with sugar attached. This blood test is not a fasting test.
- **Random blood sugar test.** A blood sample is taken at a random time, regardless of when you last ate. A random blood sugar level of 200 milligrams per deciliter (mg/dL) or higher suggests diabetes.
- **Fasting blood sugar test.** A blood sample is taken after an overnight fast. A fasting blood sugar level less than 100 mg/dL is normal. A fasting blood sugar level from 100 to 125 mg/dL is considered prediabetes. If it's 126 mg/dL or higher on two separate tests, you have diabetes.
- **Oral glucose tolerance test.** You fast overnight, and your fasting blood sugar level is measured. Then you drink a sugary liquid, and your blood sugar level is tested periodically for the next two hours. A blood sugar level less than 140 mg/dL is normal. A reading of more than 200 mg/dL after two hours indicates diabetes. A reading between 140 and 199 mg/dL indicates prediabetes.
- **Urine test.** If type 1 diabetes is suspected, your urine may be tested for ketones.

Now that you have taken tests and determined what type of diabetes is present, here are more treatments provided;

- **Diet**
- **Exercise**
- **Oral medications**
- **Insulin is the main treatment**

Healthy Alternatives

There are a wide variety of natural vitamins and minerals which can help ease the degree of diabetes as well as help control it from further complicating your health. They are;

- **Thiamine (B1)** – can limit the formation of dangerous by-products of glucose metabolism, remove oxidative stress, and improve endothelial function. May also reduce cardiovascular risk and angiopathic complications.
- **Vitamin B12** – has been shown to cause symptomatic improvement among patients with severe diabetic neuropathy and improve somatic symptoms like pain and paresthesia.
- **Vitamin C** – is an antioxidant which plays a protective role in diabetes by reducing the damage caused by free radicals. Vitamin C also improves glycosylated hemoglobin in type 2 diabetes.
- **Vitamin D** – helps improve the body's sensitivity to insulin and helps reduce the risk of insulin resistance. Vitamin D can also help lower blood sugar levels.
- **Vitamin E** – is beneficial in reducing blood glucose, inflammation, lipid peroxidation, BP, and TC levels. Vitamin E also works as an antioxidant.

- **Magnesium** – plays a huge role in the health of the human body. It also manages your insulin and carbohydrate metabolism. It helps your body's ability to secrete insulin and also help your cells use insulin more effectively. Magnesium also helps the body reduce insulin resistance.

Other minerals to consider;

- **Cinnamon** – helps lower blood sugar levels by imitating the effects of insulin and increasing glucose transport into cells. Cinnamon also helps lower blood sugar by increasing insulin sensitivity, this makes the insulin more effective with moving glucose into cells.
- **Resveratrol** – is effective in modulating blood glucose levels, decreasing insulin resistance, inhibiting chronic inflammation, improving blood lipid profiles, attenuating diabetic hypertension and countering oxidative stress. Resveratrol also helps against insulin resistance.
- **Chromium** – is known to help lower blood sugar levels and may improve insulin sensitivity and glucose metabolism.

ERECTILE DYSFUNCTION (ED)

Forgive me if I blush or even chuckle while writing about this subject matter. I admit, it is something I have dealt with a time or two in my life. So, what exactly is erectile dysfunction?

Erectile dysfunction is when a man can't get or keep an erection firm enough for sexual intercourse. It can be a bit frightening and embarrassing too. Here is a guy with a beautiful woman but yet, he can't get turned on enough to pleasure her, much less himself. I know, I know, there are other ways but we are talking about a guy's manhood. Something which has gone back in history for centuries.

While this is a serious concern for some, we need to lighten up and have a little humor with it as well. You might be surprised on how hard it is not to use the usual slang terms. You know what I am talking about. Morning wood, boner, a chubby, or straight to the point, hard-on!

There! It's out of my system! Now we can move on with it!

I suppose since I am writing about this, I will use myself as the example of erectile dysfunction to a degree. As I mentioned, I have at one time or another dealt with it and its funny the reaction I have gotten from the opposite sex. "Maybe you should see a doctor about it" or "you know, there is a pill for that"!

Did these women ever stop for a moment and consider perhaps it was them who was causing my erectile dysfunction issue? It's true! Perhaps I just wasn't all that into them. Or perhaps it was the surrounding circumstances. Maybe it was also guilt or a sense of uneasiness causing it.

We will get to those things in a minute but truthfully, unless you have been in a serious accident or have some life altering disease, erectile dysfunction is all psychological in my opinion. I know there are also some physical aspects, but I have to tell you, I just can't think of a doctor prescribing a pump as a means to getting an erection. Maybe I am off my rocker but isn't this what my partner is for?

Here is a short story of an event which eventually involved erectile dysfunction.

Imagine a friend who you have known for years and someone you found attractive but yet, questioned their choices in life. This friend wins contests at work all the time which included trips to sunny beaches and blue water. No, I was never invited to come along on the trips but one day, this friend called me up and asked if I would go with her to the casino.

Mind you, I am not the casino type. I usually just throw twenty bucks out the window as I pass by one because I know it will take me longer to find a parking space than to lose my money.

I hesitantly agreed to pick her up and drive 45 minutes to the casino. As we drove, she told me what the plan was. And it was quite an interesting plan. Her most recent paycheck before the trip wasn't as large as it should or could have been because she had missed work for personal reasons.

As we get to the casino, she informs me, her goal is to double her paycheck by playing a particular slot machine. Yes, I questioned the choice and thought, she could lose it all and then what?

She was so confident the machine was going to hit soon so she cashed her check sat down at the slot machine and began sticking twenties in the machine. I am gagging from the smoke-filled room.

As she starts playing the max bet, (thank goodness she was only playing quarter slots) I began to people watch and try to figure out everyone's story. One hour passed than another and another and she was starting to run out of money. I kept telling her the house always wins and she was putting herself in a worse set of circumstances. The story does have to do with erectile dysfunction, I promise.

We continued to sit at the machine when all of a sudden, she excuses herself mentioning a bathroom and asking me to watch the machine. Once again, I hesitantly agree to do as she asks and she is off on her way. Eventually my patience starts to wear thin as I start wondering where she is.

Just then, she shows up with more cash and a story on how she got it. Plunks it into the machine and we are on our way for the next hour as the lights flash, the bells and whistles seem to get louder but the stale smoke smell lingers. Another couple hours pass and she disappears again.

Again, returning with more money, I am starting to get physically agitated. We have been here already for 6 hours. What a total waste of time and yes, money too but I am there as a friend, not a life coach. All of a sudden, she looks at me and says, "thank you for being here with me, I will make it up to you when we get back to my place". She played out her remaining cash.

Ding Ding Ding! No, that wasn't bells going off in my head, excited because in my future I was going to get some. No, it was the machine paying out a certain amount of cash.

In fact, it paid out double of what my friend had originally came with so in her mind, she had done exactly what she came there to do, double her money. While I knew the truth, I was more excited because now we could leave!

We got back to her place and she asked me to come in for a bit.

Once again, I hesitantly agreed. Yes, I was attracted to her but there were so many factors as to why I wasn't aroused by her. We went to her room and started kissing and making out. I admit, this part was nice but then as we went further, my mind started to step in and remind me of all the reasons I needed to get out of there.

This is when the remarks mentioned early were spoken. I wasn't getting aroused and it showed. The whole mind over matter was prevalent and it just wasn't going to happen. Not after the night I experienced, not as a supposed reward, and certainly not without any partner participation. I needed to go and go is what I did. The next day she was too busy to talk as she got ready for her trip.

As our communication lessened over the weeks, months and years, we never spoke of that night ever again. Maybe it was simply two people in the wrong place at the wrong time, spending their time doing the wrong things. I truly believe my inability to get aroused was mind over matter.

Or was it?

Causes/Risk Factors

Let's get to the causes and risk factors because there are quite a few.

- **Stress** is one of the biggest culprits of ED as life is filled with responsibilities, worries about the job and money, and even stress within relationships can have a toll on the function of your penis.
- **Medications** are prescribed almost daily and as you get older chances are you have one or two medications having side-effects that affect your ability to get an erection.

- **Alcohol** has been known to put a damper on the bedroom fun do to over indulging. Other street drugs are included in this as well.

- **Depression** as part of stress can certainly have a hand in your manhood. Again, low self-esteem, low self-image plays a part in your ability to get aroused.

- **Low libido** is another erection killer and in fact, you may be done before even getting started. The lack of interest in itself is reason for concern and something which needs to be checked out.

- **Overweight** can play a big part in low self-image but also creates other factors which keep one for obtaining an erection. Chances are with indulging in food, your weight is causing your body to decrease its testosterone, causing high blood pressure and reduces blood flow to your manhood.

- **Anxiety** while connected to stress and depression can also cause the lack of arousal. There can be anxiety of the partner, the environment, and the circumstances. The mind is a powerful weapon and many times, it is used against ourselves. Learning to relax is key.

- **Anger** obviously is a mood killer and I once asked someone if getting naked during an argument with a partner would end the argument or cause even more of a situation. Seems to me getting naked would turn the focus away from anger to excitement. Being enraged whether it's regarding your partner or something completely different will never lead to a good bedroom experience.

- **Overall Health** is important to consider when one is having difficulty getting aroused and having a functioning erection. Diabetes, high blood pressure, hardening of the arteries, spinal cord injuries, and multiple sclerosis can contribute to ED.

Usual Treatments

Like in any ailment, there have been quite a few treatments tried. It's like throwing straw against a wet wall and seeing what sticks! Just the same, here are some treatments prescribed and tried:

- **Lifestyle Changes** One of the first things that is going to happen is an assessment is done to see where improvements can be made right off the bat. Whether it is diet, exercise or mental health, expect changes to be suggested.
- **Smoking & Alcohol** No, no, no! If you are a smoker or like to indulge in alcohol on a regular basis, don't come complaining about lack of stamina or sexual desire! You only have yourself to blame. Remember, you are what your body is! Better choices might be needed.
- **Exercise** Sitting on the couch shoving food or drink in your mouth is not exercise. Sitting at a desk all day too isn't helping your libido or ED problem either. You can try to exercise it all you want but if you aren't getting off your butt and doing regular exercise like walking, jogging, running, swimming, hiking or anything else to get your heart rate up, you just don't need to worry about getting your heart rate up in the bedroom. It just isn't happening!
- **Mental Health** Yes, mental health is the latest buzz word/craze but it is truly affecting your ability to get it up and satisfy your partner. Stress, anxiety, anger are just a few emotional barriers to keep you from a healthy sex life. Finding someone to talk with about the things bothering you can help immensely! A friend, psychotherapist and/or a life coach could help!
- **Medications** You can't turn on the radio or television without seeing or hearing an ad for some kind of pill that will have you satisfying your partner in no time, some-times

for hours! Good luck with that and enjoy your visit to the ER, bonehead!

It's true and it has happened quite often. Another thing you should know about. Once you start taking pills for things your body should be doing, you are in it for life. Your body will adjust to what is being digested and will start producing less and less until you are completely dependent on the little pill.

Some other types of treatment

I have to say, some of these had me scratching my head, rolling my eyes and even laughing my ass off! Yes, I said that!

- **Testosterone Therapy** – There is nothing wrong with having your testosterone checked (if they will let you) but just know one thing, once you start a testosterone therapy program, there is no turning back. Your body will stop producing testosterone all together. Yes, this is a proven fact!
- **Penis Injections (penile injections)** – Yes, this is a real thing. The injection therapy begins with Trimix, which is a mixture of 3 ingredients: alprostadil, phentolamine, and papaverine. These ingredients work by relaxing the smooth muscle and opening the blood vessels in your penis, causing an erection. Note, do not take Viagra, Levita or Stendra within 18 hours of injecting your penis or you may wish you had done so at the ER. Also, it is said you are to inject yourself 5-15 minutes before sexual intercourse! Oh, how romantic and stimulating is that?
- **Vacuum Erection Device (penis pump)** – is used to help men with erectile dysfunction get and maintain an erection. If you gotta, you gotta! Again, probably something your partner can do for you instead of a machine. Just saying!

- **Penile Implants** – are devices placed inside the penis to allow men with erectile dysfunction (ED) to get an erection. There are actually two types, semirigid and inflatable. Too bad women can't get inflatable breast implants. One size just doesn't fit all.

Okay, so I had a little fun with the other types of treatments but come on guys! There is so much more to try before you get to this point. With this said, lets get on to the next remedy, shall we?

Healthy Alternatives

Yes, healthy natural alternatives are out there and available which do work! Yes, I know this quite well. Maybe you didn't know this but some vitamin deficiencies may contribute to ED.

- **Vitamin B3 (Niacin)** can help improve cholesterol and lipid levels as well as aids in converting enzymes into energy. Vitamin B3 also helps with blood flow, which then creates a sturdier erection.
- **Vitamin B9 (Folic Acid)** acts as a mood stabilizer and helps with stress related erectile dysfunction as well as help with premature ejaculation during intercourse. It can help calm the severity of ED.
- **Vitamin C (Ascorbic Acid)** helps to improve blood flow and helps to increase testosterone levels.
- **Vitamin D** also helps improve blood to the penis and supports the production of male hormones, including testosterone.
- **L-arginine** helps relax blood vessels, allowing blood to flow freely. L-arginine can lower blood pressure too so it's good to be cautious. Also helps with heart health.

- **Citrulline** helps with blood flow, especially increasing blood flow to a man's genitals. Also helps maintain an erection.

Other minerals and herbs to consider

- **Red Ginseng (Panax)** has potential cardiovascular benefits and may reduce the risk of ED overall. Ginseng may promote the release of nitric oxide, prompting erections by relaxing the smooth muscles of the penis.
- **Horny Goat Weed (Icariin)** is an herb which has been used in China for centuries to treat low libido, erectile dysfunction, fatigue, pain, and other conditions. It also inhibits the activities of the PDE5 that is blocking dilation of the blood vessels in the penis. Also known as the natural Viagra.
- **Tongkat Ali Root Powder** may increase testosterone levels and improve male libido. Considered an aphrodisiac.

Again, before you decide to try the implants or other devices, you owe it to yourself as well as your partner to try the more natural alternatives first!

Note: I am no longer on any medication and simply rely on vitamins and supplements. I am almost 60 years old and my sex life shows no signs of slowing down any time soon!

FIBROMYALGIA

Fibromyalgia is a disorder distinguished by widespread musculoskeletal pain which is accompanied by other symptoms, including fatigue or sleep difficulties. The pain may come and go.

Causes/Risk Factors

- Women are twice as likely to have fibromyalgia than men.
- Genes passed down from parents can make you more sensitive to pain and discomfort as well as make you feel anxious or depressed, aggravating the pain.
- Lack of exercise and lack of movement can cause this condition.
- Arthritis or other infections can bring on this condition.
- Post traumatic stress disorder and other mental health illnesses can play a part in the development of fibromyalgia.
- Emotional and/or physical abuse over time can bring on this condition as the way the brain handles stress and pain changes.
- Anxiety and depression are linked to fibromyalgia as are other mood disorders.

Usual Treatments

- **Doctors & Specialists** Chances are, while you are going through exams to determine your severity with fibromyalgia, you will be seen by a rheumatologist, a doctor specializing in conditions which affect muscles and joints. Also seen by a neurologist, specializing in conditions of the central nervous system as well as a psychologist, specializing in mental health and psychological treatment.
- **Medications** There are a variety of medications that will be considered. These types of medications include pain relievers, muscle relaxers, and even some psychotic medications.
- **Counseling and Therapy** If your fibromyalgia is prompted by stress and anxiety due to emotional and physical abuse, chances are you will be assigned a counselor or a therapist specialized in your condition.
- **Lifestyle Changes Your environment and lifestyle** could be assessed and recommendations made to your lifestyle as a way to lessen the triggers which affect your fibromyalgia.

Healthy Alternatives

- **Vitamin A** helps with body pain as it helps your immune system, eye sight, reproduction and growth and development. It also helps the lungs, heart and other organs work properly.
- **Vitamin B1 (thiamin)** working as an anti-inflammatory, high doses of thiamin have shown to help improve symptoms of fibromyalgia, specifically pain.
- **Vitamin B2 (riboflavin)** is a water-soluble vitamin and helps break down proteins, fats, and carbohydrates. Riboflavin also helps convert carbohydrates into adenosine

triphosphate (ATP). The human body produces ATP from food, and ATP produces energy as the body requires it.

- **Vitamin B3 (niacin)** helps the body make various sex and stress-related hormones in the adrenal glands and other parts of the body. Niacin helps improve circulation, and it has been shown to suppress inflammation. Acts as natural pain reliever.
- **Vitamin B5 (pantothenic acid)** helps in the manufacturing of red blood cells, maintaining healthy digestive tracts and most importantly production of anti-stress hormones. Helps build energy molecules.
- **Vitamin B6 (pyridoxine)** supports the central nervous system as well as metabolism. It also helps to turn food into energy and helps with the creation of neurotransmitters, such as dopamine and serotonin which works as an anti-depressant.
- **Vitamin B7 (biotin)** helps promote appropriate function of the nervous system and is essential for liver metabolism. Biotin is commonly used to strengthen hair and nails, and in skin care. It also aids cell growth as well as helps the maintenance of mucous membranes.
- **Vitamin B9 (folate acid)** helps with proper brain function as well as playing an important role in mental and emotional well-being. B9 is also instrumental in the body's genetic material.
- **Vitamin B12 (cyanocobalamin)** plays an important role in ensuring the normal function of the brain and the central nervous system.
- **Vitamin C** acts as an antioxidant, protecting your cells from damage as well as reduces physical impairment.
- **Vitamin D** has anti-inflammatory properties which contribute to relieving pain and may alleviate other symptoms.

- **Vitamin E** can act as an antioxidant, protecting your cells from damage caused by free radicals. Vitamin E is also essential to the health of your vision, health of your blood and your immune system.
- **Turmeric** with incredible anti-inflammatory properties, turmeric helps to alleviate muscle pain and inflammation discomfort.
- **CoQ10** alleviates pain and reduces brain activity and mitochondrial dysfunction. It is also able to reduce pain and increase cognition and mood in fibromyalgia.
- **Magnesium** helps to avoid muscle spasms, weakness and back pain as well as keeping the heart, kidneys and bones healthy and strong. Getting enough magnesium can help with fatigue, sleep difficulties, and anxiety.
- **Ginger** is helpful in pain management and can ease nausea and improve digestion. Ginger can also increase antioxidant activity in the body due to its anti-inflammatory and antibacterial chemicals that are antioxidants.

HEADACHE

I just woke up with a headache! Ouch! Did I sleep wrong? Work too hard? Have some kind of illness which caused my headache? Could be, but who really knows?

I get them and I am sure you do too. The real problem is, none of the major medical institutions in this country can agree in general what a headache is and/or what causes them. Kind of like a great mystery!

One institution says a headache is this but another one says it is that. Which is it? I am getting a headache just thinking about it. So exactly, what is it?

A headache is pain or discomfort in the head, scalp, or neck. There are commonly, 3 types of headaches. They include;

- **Tension headache** – Some say a tension headache is pain across the forehead while others say it likely starts from muscle tightness in the shoulders, neck, scalp, and jaw. It may be related to stress, depression, and anxiety but also could be related to having your head and neck in an unusual position. Someone with a neck injury could also experience tension like headaches.

  This type of headache tends to start in the neck and move up and over the head to the forehead. It tends to produce a dull pain or pressure being applied to your head and neck area.

- **Migraine headaches** – Again, some say a migraine headache only occurs on one side or the other of the head while people like me who have experienced tension and migraine headaches will tell you it happens all over the head. I only wish it was one side or the other. Migraine headaches are the worst with pain that is throbbing and pulsating and even pounding at times. No matter what position you try to put your head in, there is no relief.

  Then there is the sensitivity to light and loud sounds. At times, wishing you could just pop your head off and replace it with something new and soothing. You know its bad when the nausea kicks in. You want life to just be over. "Oh, please take me already!" Yes, this is how bad they are and they can last for days.

- **Cluster Headaches** – I really feel bad for people who get cluster headaches because you guessed it, they come in clusters. Several very painful headaches a day and this can go on for months. Then all of a sudden, they are gone for weeks/months and some don't ever get them again. Like I said, headaches are a great mystery!

Another type of headache is a sinus headache which occurs due to swelling in the sinus cavity and passages behind the eyes, nose and cheeks. The pain is in the front of head and face and is even worse when you bend over. So don't bend over!

Causes/Risk Factors

While there are several known risk factors, actual causes are still being studied. Some of the risk factors are as follows;

- **Colds**, a fever, the flu and/or premenstrual syndrome.
- **Temporal Arteritis** – A swollen, inflamed artery which supplies blood to the neck, temple and different parts of the head.
- **Hypertension** – High blood pressure can be a sign of underlying health issues but, certainly contributes to the frequency of headaches.
- **Brain Tumor** – growths inside the head/brain can cause headaches.
- **Dizziness** – Again, perhaps a sign of an underlying health issue but it can lead to headaches.
- **Brain Swelling** – The build up of fluid inside the skull.
- **Brain Infections** such as meningitis, encephalitis, or other bacterial infections.
- **Sleep Apnea** – Lack of oxygen during sleep
- **Dehydration** – Not keeping hydrated with water is a sure cause for headaches.

Usual Treatments

- **Relaxations techniques** – Finding a quiet place to rest and try to clear the mind.
- **Cool cloth** – A cool cloth soothes the forehead as well as relaxes the brain.
- **Sleep** – Getting the recommended 8 hours of sleep daily goes a long way to alleviating the probability of getting headaches.
- **Medications** – Medications are prescribed to help with pain relief and other effects of the headache or underlying health issues.

Other Treatments:

CT Scan, MRI, x-rays, and blood pressure monitoring.

Healthy Alternatives

- **Vitamin B2 (riboflavin)** is a water-soluble vitamin that helps break down proteins, fats, and carbohydrates. Riboflavin also helps convert carbohydrates into adenosine triphosphate (ATP). The human body produces ATP from food, and ATP produces energy as the body requires it.
- **Vitamin B3 (niacin)** helps the body make various sex and stress-related hormones in the adrenal glands and other parts of the body. Niacin helps improve circulation, and it has been shown to suppress inflammation. Acts as natural pain reliever.
- **Vitamin D** has anti-inflammatory properties which contribute to relieving pain and may alleviate other symptoms.
- **CoQ10** alleviates pain and reduces brain activity and mitochondrial dysfunction. It is also able to reduce pain and increase cognition and mood in fibromyalgia.
- **Magnesium** helps to avoid muscle spasms, weakness and pain as well as keeping the heart, kidneys and bones healthy and strong. Getting enough magnesium can help with fatigue, sleep difficulties, and anxiety.
- **Ginger** is helpful in pain management and can ease nausea and improve digestion. Ginger can also increase antioxidant activity in the body due to its anti-inflammatory and antibacterial chemicals that are antioxidants.
- **Melatonin** helps signal the brain that it is time for sleep as it is reported that lack of sleep contributes to migraines.

- **Lavender Oil** is used to treat pain and boost mood. Also helps reduce stress hormones.
- **Menthol** has a calming effect as well as cooling effect when rubbed on the neck and forehead.

Please do not stop taking your prescribed medications like I did without consulting your care provider first.

High Blood Pressure (Hypertension)

High blood pressure occurs when the pressure against the blood vessel walls in your body is consistently too high. While most medical authorities will say high blood pressure has no symptoms, I beg to differ. I believe headaches, blurred vision, and pain in the chest are pretty good signs of high blood pressure and other underlying health issues.

This is just my opinion and while I am not a doctor, I am an authority on my high blood pressure and the other blood pressure related conditions I have experienced.

Causes/Risk Factors

While it is said there are no real symptoms for high blood pressure, there are certainly many risk factors, including;

- **Age** causes arteries to stiffen, called arteriosclerosis or hardening of the arteries. This is normal with growing older.
- **Environment** is another factor as working around toxins can put you at greater risk. Having a lot of stress at work, sitting for long periods of time, and interrupted sleep patterns place greater stress on your body.

- **Genetics** is something you can't take for granted. Finding out your family health history can go a long way in avoiding trouble and even preventing CAD further down the road.
- **Physical Inactivity** can worsen other heart related risk factors such as high blood pressure, high blood cholesterol, obesity, and diabetes.
- **Smoking or even second-hand smoke** can lead to health issues which puts a lot of stress on your heart.
- **Diet and Lifestyle** have a huge impact on your health and can be the difference between a healthy life or that of heart related chronic illness.
- **Race and Ethnicity** plays a big part in the people who experience coronary heart disease. CAD is the leading cause of death for people of most racial and ethnic groups in the United States, including African Americans. For Hispanics, Asian Americans or Pacific Islanders, and American Indians or Alaska Natives, heart disease is second only to cancer.
- **Gender** also plays a role as to when one can expect to deal with heart related issues. Coronary heart disease affects men and women while obstructive coronary artery disease is more common in men. Non-obstructive coronary disease is more common in women. In men, the risk for coronary heart disease starts to increase around age 45 while women have a lower risk of coronary heart disease until around the age of 55.

Usual Treatments

- **Lifestyle Change** – Changing diet by decreasing salt (sodium) intake.
- **Weight Loss** – Consider losing weight and/or maintaining a healthy weight. This will help relieve stress.

- **Become Active** – By increasing your activity such as exercising, you can help your health in a number of ways, including lowering blood pressure, lowering bad cholesterol, and simply make you feel better all around.
- **Smoking and Alcohol** – Decrease and/or eliminating smoking and alcohol all together will have instant benefits and help lower your high blood pressure.
- **Managing Stress** – While it can depend on your life circumstances, finding ways to lower and maintain your stress will go a long way to helping keep your blood pressure in check. Perhaps a change in career is needed, or eliminating those who cause you stress.

High blood pressure is also considered a symptom of heart disease, which may lead to other tests and treatments.

Healthy Alternatives

- **Vitamin C** acts as an antioxidant, protecting your cells from damage as well as reducing physical impairment. Vitamin C also acts as a diuretic, helping to remove excess fluid from your body, helping to lower the pressure inside your blood vessels.
- **Vitamin E** can act as an antioxidant, protecting your cells from damage caused by free radicals. Vitamin E is also essential to the health of your vision, health of your blood and your immune system. It also contains nitric oxide which can improve blood pressure levels.
- **CoQ10** alleviates pain and reduces brain activity and mitochondrial dysfunction. It is also able to reduce pain and increase cognition and mood in fibromyalgia.
- **Magnesium** helps to avoid muscle spasms, weakness and back pain as well as keeping the heart, kidneys and bones

healthy and strong. Getting enough magnesium can help with fatigue, sleep difficulties, and anxiety.

- **L-arginine** helps relax blood vessels, allowing blood to flow freely. L-arginine can lower blood pressure too so it's good to be cautious. Also helps with heart health.
- **Potassium** helps relax the pressure within the blood vessels as well as helping to lower sodium levels which can help reduce blood pressure.
- **Omega 3** – is good for heart health as it contains both docosahexaenoic acid (DHA) and eicosapentaenoic acid (EPA). This can help unclog arteries and can reduce levels of blood fat called triglyceride.
- **Selenium** – antioxidant activity of selenium helps control blood pressure and may even help prevent hypertension. Selenium can help lower inflammation and oxidative stress of the body.
- **Calcium** – increased use of calcium has shown to lower blood pressure and help bring it down to a normal level. It also helps blood vessels relax, alleviating pressure.

High Cholesterol

High cholesterol is when you have too much of a fatty substance in your blood, which may limit blood flow, increasing the risk of heart attack or stroke.

There are two main types of cholesterol;

LDL (low-density lipoprotein), "bad" cholesterol, makes up most of your body's cholesterol particles. These particles build up within the walls of arteries, causing them to become hard and narrow.

HDL (high-density lipoprotein), "good" cholesterol, absorbs excess cholesterol and carries it back to the liver.

While there are technically no symptoms for high cholesterol, some consider a symptom of high blood pressure, heart attacks, diabetes, chest pain, stroke as well as other pains throughout the body. **Cholesterol levels are determined by a blood test.**

Causes/Risk Factors

Many different lifestyle factors can contribute to high blood cholesterol, including;

- **Unhealthy diet** – consuming too much saturated fat or trans fat contributes to high cholesterol.

- **Smoking** – makes your LDL "bad" cholesterol 'adhesive' – so it clings to your artery walls and clogs them up easier while lowering your levels of HDL "good" cholesterol, which normally takes cholesterol away from the artery walls.
- **Lack of exercise** – there are plenty of studies which have connected the dots between lack of exercise and adverse health conditions. High cholesterol doesn't escape this either. In fact, it has been proven quite the opposite.
- **Underlying condition** – such as high blood pressure, diabetes and heart disease.

Other factors include;

- **Age** – your body's metabolism changes as you age. While unhealthy cholesterol levels can be detected at any age, most people between 40 and 59 years of age are diagnosed with high cholesterol. The liver has a harder time eliminating "bad" cholesterol as we age.
- **Genes** – Family history is a good indicator on whether you will develop high cholesterol as well as other diseases as genes can be passed from one generation to another.
- **Race and Ethnicity** – this is an area or factor which caused me to scratch my head a bit. Particularly number 4.
  1. Overall, non-Hispanic white people are more likely than other groups to have high levels of total cholesterol.
  2. Asian Americans, including those of Indian, Filipino, Japanese, and Vietnamese descent, are more likely to have high levels of "bad" LDL cholesterol than other groups.
  3. Hispanic Americans are more likely to have lower levels of "good" HDL cholesterol than other groups.
  4. African Americans are more likely than other groups to

have high levels of "good" HDL cholesterol. However, they are more likely to have other risk factors, such as high blood pressure, obesity, or diabetes, which may overcome the health benefit of higher HDL levels.

- **Sex** – Women's risk of high cholesterol goes up after menopause as it lowers levels of female hormones which help protect a woman from high cholesterol. Men have a higher risk of high cholesterol then women from age 20 to 39 years of age.
- **Medications** – some medicines taken for other health issues can raise your level of "bad" LDL cholesterol or lower your level of "good" HDL cholesterol. They include;
  1. Arrhythmia medicines
  2. Beta-blockers for relieving angina chest pain or treating high blood pressure
  3. Chemotherapy medicines used to treat cancer
  4. Diuretics to treat high blood pressure
  5. Immunosuppressive medicines to treat inflammatory diseases or to prevent rejection after organ transplant
  6. Retinoids to treat acne
  7. Steroids to treat inflammatory diseases such as lupus, rheumatoid arthritis, and psoriasis

Usual Treatments

Healthy Diet – is the primary treatment to high cholesterol. Trying to eat better foods and reduce saturated fats and eliminate trans fats. Consuming whey protein and increasing soluble fiber.

Exercise – yes, exercise, exercise, and exercise! Exercising stimulates enzymes which move LDL from the blood and blood vessel walls to the liver. Moderate physical activities can help raise HDL levels.

Medications – Statins are usually prescribed to help lower "bad" cholesterol and raise "good" cholesterol levels over time. Usually takes 3-6 months to see a real change.

Healthy Alternatives

- **Vitamin B3 (niacin)** increases the level of good cholesterol and reduces triglycerides, another fat which can clog arteries. Niacin helps improve circulation, and it has been shown to suppress inflammation.
- **Vitamin B12 (cyanocobalamin)** can lower cholesterol naturally, but also provide additional cardiovascular health benefits which plays an important role in ensuring the normal function of the brain and the central nervous system.
- **Vitamin C** reduces LDL "bad") cholesterol and blood triglycerides. Also acts as an antioxidant, protecting your cells from damage as well as reducing the risk of heart disease.
- **Vitamin D** seems to have an effect on reducing serum total cholesterol, LDL cholesterol, and triglyceride levels but not HDL cholesterol levels. Also has anti-inflammatory properties which contribute to relieving pain and may alleviate other symptoms.
- **Vitamin E** can act as an antioxidant, protecting your cells from damage caused by free radicals. Vitamin E is also essential to the health of your vision, health of your blood and your immune system.
- **Turmeric** is beneficial against high cholesterol because it contains a compound called curcumin. Curcumin has been proven to lower LDL cholesterol and prevent its oxidation, suppressing plaque build-up in arteries.

- **CoQ10** has been shown to help the heart in many ways. It can reduce low-density lipoprotein "bad" cholesterol, lower blood pressure, and lower the risk of a heart attack.
- **Magnesium** studies have shown increased intake of magnesium may lower blood triglyceride level and increase high-density lipoprotein (HDL) cholesterol level.
- **Ginger** is helpful in lowering your total cholesterol and triglycerides levels while increasing HDL cholesterol levels.
- **Zinc** significantly reduces total cholesterol, LDL cholesterol and triglycerides.

Please do not stop taking your prescribed medications like I did without consulting your care provider first.

MENOPAUSE

Menopause is the natural biological process in women which attributes to the end of menstruation, usually 12 months after the last period. Once a woman begins menopause, she stops producing eggs, meaning her years of reproducing naturally are over. She can still get pregnant however with a doner egg.

There are 3 stages of menopause and they include;

- **Perimenopause** – your menstrual cycle becomes irregular and most women start to experience this in the mid to late forties.
- **Menopause** – at this stage, you have had your last menstrual period.
- **Postmenopause** – occurs 12 months after your last and final period.

Causes/Risk Factors

- Declining reproductive hormones
- Primary ovarian function insufficiency
- Chemotherapy/radiation therapy
- Surgery (oophorectomy) removes ovaries.

Symptoms

- Irregular periods
- Chills
- Sleep issues
- Night sweats
- Vaginal dryness
- Weight gain
- Mood swings
- Slowed metabolism

Usual Treatments

While symptoms are enough to tell when a woman is going through the stages of menopause, there are also blood tests conducted for different circumstances. These tests are;

- **Thyroid stimulating hormone (TSH)** – to check how well your thyroid is working as an underactive thyroid can create signs and symptoms of menopause (hypothyroidism).
- **Follicle stimulating hormone (FSH) and estrogen (estradiol)** – measures your increase in FSH levels and decrease of estradiol levels as menopause occurs.
- **Hormone therapy** – such as estrogen therapy, helps to protect against the thinning of bone such as osteoporosis as well as helps ease vaginal dryness symptoms associated with menopause.
- **Lifestyle changes** – the usual change of diet, exercising, prescribed medications, and avoiding the things which seem to cause your symptoms to flare up.

Healthy Alternatives

- **Vitamin A** supports vision, immunity and thyroid function as well as helps with hormone chances by lessening the stress and supporting thyroid function.
- **Vitamin B6** has been shown to help with menopausal depression and increase energy by boosting serotonin. B6 is also needed to optimize metabolism, manage inflammation and boost the immune system.
- **Vitamin B12** is essential for the formation of red blood cells and is a key component for increasing energy. Helps support vision, gut health, the heart, brain and central nervous system. Can also help reduce insomnia and hot flashes.
- **Vitamin C** helps lessen hot flashes and is an important component for bone density. It is also an antioxidant and fights against heart disease.
- **Vitamin D** helps build strong bones supports the proper function of muscles, supports neurological function, immune system, and helps regulate blood sugar.
- **Vitamin K** is another vitamin which helps build and protect bone density but also helps prevent blood clots. Vitamin K also boosts blood vessel health.
- **Magnesium** is important for improving heart health, reducing blood pressure, decreasing risk of diabetes, combatting osteoporosis, and particularly if you take magnesium citrate, easing constipation—all issues which increase with menopause. Also helps with calming anxiety, easing joint pain, improving sleep and hot flashes
- **Calcium** is an important mineral that women need more of as estrogen levels decline. Also helps keep muscles working properly as well as supports the central nervous system.

- **Omega 3** helps keep triglyceride levels where they need to be and helps to decrease depression and hot flashes. Omega 3 is also good for heart health but may also thin blood.
- **Probiotics** are essential to good gut health. You have trillions of microorganisms inside your body and gut, doing good things like helping you digest, supporting mental health, and supporting physiological function.
- **Turmeric** has anti-inflammatory properties, boosts heart health and helps to relieve depression. Also acts as an anti-coagulant.

Multiple Sclerosis (MS)

A disease which impacts the brain, spinal cord, and optical nerves. A disease where the immune system attacks the protective cover of nerve components (myelin), axons and neurons, destroying the body's central nervous system. MS affects more women than men and the diagnosis is usually determined between the age of 20 and 40.

I have seen first hand how MS can take away a person's ability to do the simplest functions we take for granted on a daily basis. I know a special man who if not for his diagnosis of MS 30 plus years ago, would have continued to work well into his sixties, but would still be an avid hunter, golfer, fisherman, and bowler. The thought of this disease skipping generations scares me to no end and will always have me concerned for my children.

Causes/Risk Factors

While the cause of multiple sclerosis is unknown, it is an auto-immune disease which causes the immune system to malfunction in the way it was intended to function. Symptoms include but are not limited to;

- **Vision loss** – is one of the early signs of the disease. Some people even have their vision restored, fooling medical professionals to think it is something else altogether.
- **Loss of coordination** – simple steps are a struggle and can even result in being wheelchair bound as you begin to lose strength and control.
- **Fatigue** – MS causes a person to become fatigued due to the struggle and exertion.
- **Pain** – because the immune system attacks and eats away the protective fatty substance which coats nerve fibers, it leaves the nerves exposed and causes miscommunication between the brain, spinal cord and the body's nervous system.
- **Loss of bladder function** – MS destroys your senses as well as creates miscommunication with the brain and other bodily functions.
- **Memory issues** – MS can affect long term/short term memory.
- **Sexual difficulties** – Unable to function in a sexual manner as well as eventually losing interest altogether.

Usual Treatments

Again, while there is no cure for MS, most treatment consists of treating symptoms.

Medications – which suppress the immune system and help with spasms as well as pain. Anti-inflammatory drugs are also used as is chemotherapy and steroids. Botox is beginning to become a drug of choice, helping calm nerves.

Physical therapy – Working with muscle memory and keeping joints in working condition.

Mental health – consists of attending a group gathering with other MS patients, attending counseling, and working with neuropsychologist to help cope with disease.

Other treatments considered

Many MS patients are desperate enough to try and recover a normal portion of their lives that they subject themselves to more controversial treatments such as;

- **Bee stings** – it is suggested that this benefits people with a range of MS, because bee stings cause inflammation, leading to an anti-inflammatory reaction of the immune system. More studies are needed.
- **Liberation therapy (Venoplasty)** – involves opening up narrowed veins from the brain and spinal cord due to a condition of compromised blood flow in return veins from the central nervous system. Many claims have since been discredited.

Healthy Alternatives

- **Vitamin A** helps with body pain as it helps your immune system, eyesight, reproduction and growth and development. It also helps the lungs, heart and other organs work properly.
- **Vitamin B5 (pantothenic acid)** helps in the manufacturing of red blood cells, maintaining healthy digestive tracts and most importantly production of anti-stress hormones. Helps build energy molecules.
- **Vitamin B6 (pyridoxine)** supports the central nervous system as well as metabolism. It also helps to turn food into energy and helps with the creation of neurotransmitters,

such as dopamine and serotonin which works as an anti-depressant.

- **Vitamin B12 (cyanocobalamin)** plays an important role in ensuring the normal function of the brain and the central nervous system.
- **Vitamin C** acts as an antioxidant, protecting your cells from damage as well as reducing physical impairment.
- **Vitamin D** has anti-inflammatory properties which contribute to relieving pain and may alleviate other symptoms.
- **Vitamin E** can act as an antioxidant, protecting your cells from damage caused by free radicals. Vitamin E is also essential to the health of your vision, health of your blood and your immune system.
- **Magnesium** helps to avoid muscle spasms, weakness and back pain as well as keeping the heart, kidneys and bones healthy and strong. Getting enough magnesium can help with fatigue, sleep difficulties, and anxiety.
- **Ginger** is helpful in pain management and can ease nausea and improve digestion. Ginger can also increase antioxidant activity in the body due to its anti-inflammatory and antibacterial chemicals which are antioxidants.
- **Selenium** – antioxidant activity of selenium helps control blood pressure and may even help prevent hypertension. Selenium can help lower inflammation and oxidative stress of the body.
- **Calcium** is an important mineral which women need more of as estrogen levels decline. Also helps keep muscles working properly as well as supports the central nervous system.
- **Zinc** – While zinc is good for us, it seems to get mixed results in studies when it comes to multiple sclerosis. Some say it's the zinc deficiency which contributes to MS while

other studies find that high levels of zinc may worsen symptoms as it stimulates the immune system.

Other alternatives

- **St. John's Wort** – is known to help with depression, a symptom many MS patients struggle with. Be sure to talk with your physician before taking St. John's wort as it has been known to interact with medications.
- **Asian Ginseng** – increases energy in the body and may contribute to easing some of the symptoms of MS like fatigue. It is also used for increasing strength and boosting the immune system. Again, don't take without consulting your primary care provider.
- **Echinacea** – has been linked to shortening colds and other viral respiratory infections as well as helping to make these symptoms and infections less severe.
- **Ginkgo Biloba** – Another Chinese herb linked to lessening fatigue in people suffering from MS. Beware though, Ginkgo Biloba doesn't interact kindly with many medications.
- **Valerian** – a herb native to Europe and parts of Asia which helps with sleep as well as reducing anxiety.

Note: The herbs listed above, can have beneficial components for the body and your health, they can also have adverse reactions when mixed with other medications. Always do your research and consult your primary care provider before consumption.

Please do not stop taking your prescribed medications like I did without consulting your care provider first.

OBESITY/OTHER WEIGHT ISSUES

When I was 23 and just out of the Army, I could walk into Mc Donald's, order a Big Mac meal, 20-piece chicken nuggets and eventually go back for another cheeseburger without batting an eye. I figured I was in shape, was pretty active, and my metabolism was still burning at a high level.

About three years later, I felt a shift in my body and also in my activity. While I was still pretty active working and hanging out with friends, I was also spending a lot of time in the bars drinking. It wasn't until I saw my engagement pictures that I began to realize something was wrong. I didn't look good at all. In fact, I looked like the "Pillsbury doughboy" from the commercials on tv.

I was shocked when I saw the pictures but was surprised that I hadn't noticed it in the mirror every time I got out of the shower. Was it avoidance or did it happen over time and I just became use to it? Perhaps I just thought this was how life goes, enjoy your early 20s because after which, real life sets in.

Nope, I wasn't buying it! I mean, I graduated from high school a hundred and thirty-five pounds. I also had left the military weighing a hundred and forty-two pounds but yet, a few years later, I was scaling a hundred and eighty-nine pounds and let me tell you, it wasn't muscle weight, it was Mc Donald's Big Mac weight! I was horrified! How did I let this happen?

Christmas Miracle

December 1989, I was hired as a mail handler with the postal service, working the night shift on the dock, unloading and sorting mail bags of different weight. It was just what the doctored ordered, well sort of. I would begin at 11:00 o'clock pm and start out on the dock.

Mind you, winters in Wisconsin were freezing and you got it, those semi-trailers had either traveled in the cold or sat in the cold for hours so they were, COLD!

My first 5 hours of work was to help upload the mail bags onto the conveyer belt and/or sort the bags at the other end onto carts we called "trucks" for the different cities the mail was going to. Here we are, battling the freezing cold, trying to stay warm and handling mail bags which weighed up to 75-pounds! Yeah right! More like a hundred and twenty-five pounds.

Needless to say, it was quite the nightly workout, 6-days a week. In the first few weeks, the blubber became my best friend. Every chance I got I was sucking down water. After about a month, I noticed my clothes feeling different and realized, I was losing the excess weight I had put on.

Again, when you work nights and have no idea what time in the morning you will get off, your eating habits suck! Some mornings it was 8:30am, others it was 10:30am and even later some days. I would go home and get to sleep just to wake up and go back to work again. Yet, I was losing weight.

I wasn't just losing weight; I was also building muscle and it was starting to show. In the first 5 weeks I lost a total of 38 pounds! Went from "Pillsbury Doughboy" to looking pretty darn good! From 189 pounds to 151 pounds! I was back to turning heads! Woo hoo! Feeling good, looking good and the confidence level was through the roof. The job still sucked but I felt great!

Most guys had to go to the gym to get my results and they certainly weren't getting them in 5 short weeks, but I was. The post office dock became my gym. Yes, I would go to a local hotel and swim a few days a week, too, after work. It was an amazing transformation.

It's interesting how the mail volume falls off after Christmas and it was all about bulk mail the next few months. Semi-trailers weren't as full as they were pre-Christmas and as it warmed up, hours at work lessened as well. At the time of my hire, I was a part-time flexible. Meaning, they would take hours away from me to give to the full-time guys just to stay full-time guys.

Another guy was hired the same time as me but because he was called first, he was given seniority over me. Then he got promoted to full-time and I began to have an attitude, calling in sick and heading to the bars again. I wasn't the star employee and my attitude was becoming substandard. To make matters worse, I could tell the weight was coming back on again too!

Eventually, I was transferred to another city, a new opportunity to make a good impression. I tried; I really did! I liked my supervisors and made a point to work hard for them. I was no longer on the docks but, actually canceling mail. The problem was, you stand in one spot for hours and I became bored.

I would start sneaking food onto the floor to snack on while working. I eventually got promoted to full-time but still wasn't happy. I started wondering off the job, going to different areas of the workplace. Acting like I was in charge and on a mission whenever someone asked me what I was up to. Eventually, I got hurt. I damaged my left shoulder and was on worker's comp for a while.

When you are on worker's comp, you work in an area where damaged mail comes to but also, it is in an area where all your co-workers come by for breaks and lunch which then led to a lot of harassment. Again, I turned to eating as my coping mechanism.

It could have been worse. I could have started drinking and taking drugs. I saw it happen on the job.

Eventually, I was let go because I copped an attitude again and stopped going to work. Crazy, I know but I saw people who worked there, working 60 to 80 hour work weeks, making a ton of money but they all looked pale and gray! They had no life and I needed to have a life, so I thought.

The roller coaster weight begins

Maybe we should actually call it the yo yo weight experience. Yep, I think so! It's funny how I would get heavy, find a way to lose it for a while then gain what I lost plus more. I went from looking like crap at 189 pounds to looking great at 151 pounds.

Then I shot up to 206 pounds, got it back down to 184 pounds, looking fabulous again and before I knew it, I had shot back up to 215 and then eventually up to 228 pounds! Yikes! Yes, it took several years to put the weight back on but I was disgusted with how I looked. Don't even get me started on how I felt. Then the bypass surgery and ruptured appendix happened.

I got back down to 188 pounds but looked sick! How was that possible? When I got down to 184-pound 6 years earlier, I looked amazing and now at 188, I looked sick? The weird thing is, something clicked in my head, making me think I needed to add weight to try not to look sick. How sick is that? Eventually, I got back up to the 215 and 228 before realizing I was killing myself.

I was now obese! Didn't matter how I looked at it, I was fat. Friends kept telling me I didn't need to lose weight and I looked good. Not great, but good! What the heck? It's my body, if I want to lose some weight and tone up, encourage me, support me but don't tell me I don't need to lose weight. It's counterproductive.

At 5'8" and 215 pounds, my body mass index (BMI) was 30.0 which is considered obese. The good news is I am not morbidly obese. Time to celebrate, right? Yeah, not so much! Even at 184 pounds, where I looked really good, I was still considered overweight with a 25.0 BMI score. In order to be in the healthy range, I have to weigh in at about 160 pounds.

If I was still 215 pounds, I would need to have lost 55 pounds in order to get to the top of the scale for a healthy BMI. Talk about ridiculous! Don't get me wrong, when I was at 184 pounds and looking good, I knew there was still room for improvement and losing another 10-15 pounds was doable.

Let's take a closer look at BMI and how it relates to obesity. A starting running back is 5'9" and is all muscle. He weighs in at 209 pounds. Wouldn't he be considered obese too? He would with just inputting the simple numbers. So why even consider or worry about your BMI?

So, what is obesity?

Obesity is a disorder which involves excessive body fat that also contributes to other health problems such as heart disease, high blood pressure and even diabetes. As mentioned above, BMI determines your number and category based on weight divided by height squared. This is an estimate of your body fat. Therefore, an athlete such as mentioned above, might fall into the obese category even though they are in great shape and have very little body fat.

Even though obesity can be genetic and influenced by hormones, most personal trainers, nutritionists and dieticians will tell you its all about the calories in and the calories out. If you are eating foods with a lot of calories but your activity level is that of a snail, chances are, you will gain weight which could result in a high BMI and you labeled as OBESE!

Causes/Risk Factors

- **Unhealthy diet** – obesity is the result of a poor diet. One which lacks vegetables and fruit, but is high in trans-fats as well as saturated fats. Another area to be concerned with is eating too much because your portion sizes are too big. Also, drinking high calory beverages will contribute to your poor health and cause you to gain weight.
- **Inactivity** – If you have a sedentary lifestyle, you will more than likely find yourself overweight. Lack of movement and/or exercise will not only keep the weight from burning off, it will eventually be hard on your joints, digestive system and your heart. A walk for 10 minutes has a tremendous amount of benefits to your body.
- **Dehydration** – Your body is made up of 75% water but yet quite often, the body gets dehydrated. This can be caused by the foods you eat and the types of beverages you are consuming. Most people do not drink as much water as they should each day.
- **Genetics** – can affect the way your body stores fat and how it is released. It also has a role in how your body converts food into energy.
- **Sleep deprivation** – the body needs sleep in order to function properly. It is just as important to the body as is food and water. Lack of sleep may contribute to the body storing more fat.
- **Medications** – If you are taking a thyroid medication, most likely you are retaining water which is contributing to your weight gain.

Usual Treatments

Lifestyle changes – There are three key areas which need to be addressed and they usually are;

- **Dietary changes** – after an assessment, you will be given a plan to help you to lose weight and become healthier. These plans usually include types of foods to eat, portion sizes as well as limiting calory intake. Calory intake for a woman trying to lose weight is usually 1,200-1,500 calories, while a man trying to lose weight is 1,500-1,800 calories. Remember, calories in minus calories out equals either weight loss or weight gain.

- **Exercise and activities** – it is recommended that we all exercise up to 150 minutes a week just to stay healthy or status quo. This physical exercise/activity needs to be moderately-intensive, especially if you want to lose weight. It is recommended that those looking to lose weight should more than double their exercise while maintaining the recommended calory intake or even taken a deficient calory count.

- **Medications** – There are medications to help suppress your appetite or to block the digestion and absorption of fat into your digestive system as well as laxatives to help move food along the digestive system.

- **Behavior changes** – our emotions have power over us and in order to change this, we need to be conscious about our habits and activities. We need to recognize our habits and know how to step in when we notice we are doing something which contributes to our weight gain or hinders our ability to lose the excess weight.

- **Counseling and Hypnosis** – Support groups are established to allow individual the opportunity to talk with and share experiences with other like-minded people within a controlled and safe environment. Hypnosis is another option when it comes to weight loss. Allowing the subconscious mind to be rewired so to speak, to either dull the taste of food even making certain foods look uninviting to the individual who desires it.

- **Surgery** – There are several types of surgery which a doctor can prescribe if he feels you would benefit from it. These surgeries include Gastric bypass surgery, Gastric sleeve, Biliopancreatic diversion with duodenal switch and Laparoscopic adjustable gastric band.

Healthy Alternatives

- **Vitamin B1 (thiamin)** works to help metabolize carbohydrates, fats, and proteins, activating stored energy instead of letting it turn to fat.
- **Vitamin B3 (niacin)** helps the body make various sex and stress-related hormones in the adrenal glands and other parts of the body. Niacin helps improve circulation, and it has been shown to suppress inflammation. Acts as a natural pain reliever.
- **Potassium** – helps relax the pressure within the blood vessels as well as helping to lower sodium levels which can help reduce blood pressure.
- **Vitamin B5 (pantothenic acid)** helps in the manufacturing of red blood cells, maintaining healthy digestive tracts and most importantly production of anti-stress hormones. Helps build energy molecules.
- **Vitamin B6 (pyridoxine)** supports the central nervous system as well as metabolism. It also helps to turn food into energy and helps with the creation of neurotransmitters,

such as dopamine and serotonin which works as an anti-depressant.

- **Vitamin B12 (cyanocobalamin)** plays an important role in ensuring the normal function of the brain and the central nervous system.
- **Vitamin C** acts as an antioxidant, protecting your cells from damage as well as reduce physical impairment.
- **Vitamin D** has anti-inflammatory properties which contribute to relieving pain and may alleviate other symptoms.
- **Calcium** is an important mineral which women need more of as estrogen levels decline. Also helps keep muscles working properly as well as supports the central nervous system.
- **CoQ10** alleviates pain and reduces brain activity and mitochondrial dysfunction. It is also able to reduce pain and increase cognition and mood in fibromyalgia.
- **Magnesium** helps to avoid muscle spasms, weakness and back pain as well as keeping the heart, kidneys and bones healthy and strong. Getting enough magnesium can help with fatigue, sleep difficulties, and anxiety.
- **Iron** is an important mineral which can help with weight loss by helping to deliver oxygen to muscles, which helps them to function. It also helps with muscle growth. Lack of iron can create low-energy and weakness.

These also improve metabolism to assist your weight loss:

- **Green tea** – Caffeine and catechins in green tea and other products may help with weight management.
- **Resveratrol** – This compound, found in the skin of red grapes, mulberries, peanuts, and more, may help burn fat. It thins the blood and keeps blood pressure in check. It

might slow blood clotting as well. Resveratrol helps reduce low-density lipoprotein (LDL) cholesterol (the "bad" cholesterol) and potentially help prevent damage to blood vessels. Helps with blood circulation.

- **Capsaicin** – fire up your metabolism with spicy treats to burn up to 50 extra calories per day.
- **Turmeric** – Curcumin, a compound in turmeric, is an antioxidant renowned for its anti-inflammatory properties and ability to boost metabolism. Turmeric also helps maintain brain function, fight chronic illnesses from cancer to heart disease, and much more.

Another quick fun weight loss story

Several years ago, I needed a physical but my long-time primary care provider was moving to a different department and I needed to find a new doctor.

Once I found one, I scheduled my physical. I show up at the time and date, go through the usual stuff until the doctor says "Okay, now we need to talk about your weight". I was like "yes, I know we do but I was wondering, what is the weight I should be at?" He goes on to tell me "You should weigh what you weighed when you graduated from high school".

My response was "Ha, that's not going to happen, I weighed 135 pounds when I graduated from high school". He then goes on to say "well, the chart says you should weight 142". Again, my response was "ha, that's not going to happen". Then the doctor asked me, "what do you think your ideal weight should be?"

"175-180?" I replied. His next sentence was "lets try for 175'! Needless to say, I never went back to him until I needed to take my son into urgent care for a broken finger. The doctor looked at me and said, "aren't you one of my patients too?" I replied with "not since our discussion about weight loss". He looked puzzled so I explained it all to him.

Then he looks at me and says while patting his own stomach, "I don't think I was or am in the right frame of health myself to be telling anyone what weight they need to be at." We have been friends ever since!

Please do not stop taking your prescribed medications like I did without consulting your care provider first.

PERIPHERAL NEUROPATHY

Peripheral neuropathy is when nerves in the body's extremities, such as the hands, feet and arms, are damaged. Usually this becomes long term and is described as painful numbness and tingling in hands, electric/shock-like pain on the sides of feet as well as muscle cramps and aches. Weakness has also been reported.

Causes/Risk Factors

Causes include diabetes, infections, injuries, alcohol abuse, low vitamin B levels, some autoimmune disorders, and poor circulation. It has been reported that chemotherapy is also related to the symptoms of peripheral neuropathy.

Symptoms regularly reported have been;

- **Numbness and tingling** – usually occurring in hands and feet and can spread upward into arms and legs.
- **Pain** – sharp jabbing pain as well as extreme burning sensations are felt in the affected areas.
- **Muscle weakness** – when motor nerves are affected, it can cause lack of coordination and falling.
- **Extreme touch sensitivity** – being more sensitive to touch or pressure.

- **Sensitivity to environment** – when you are more intolerant and sensitive to cold or hot.
- **Bowel, bladder or digestive problems** – constipation, weak bladder as well as irritable bowel are all associated with peripheral neuropathy.
- **Dizziness and lightheadedness** – caused by changes in blood pressure due to peripheral neuropathy.
- **Trouble passing urine** – hesitation and urge to go sensation are also related.
- **Trouble swallowing** – a scary sensation when you feel as though food/drink is caught in your throat is a possible sign of peripheral neuropathy.

Usual Treatments

- **Steroids** – for short-term while long term plan is created and implemented.
- **Medications** – anti-depressants and pain medication can be prescribed to help with the anxiety of symptoms.
- **Physical therapy** – is used to get motions and dexterity back in hands.
- **Relaxation therapy** – yoga, meditation and hypnosis are used for pain management as well as relaxation.
- **Acupuncture** – used to relieve pressure on the nerves in hands and feet.
- **Lifestyle changes** – balanced diet, exercising 30-60 minutes daily as well as avoiding situations which worsen nerve damage.

Healthy Alternatives

- **Vitamin A** helps with body pain as it helps your immune system, eyesight, reproduction, growth and development. It also helps the lungs, heart and other organs work properly.
- **Vitamin B1 (thiamin)** working as an anti-inflammatory, high doses of thiamin have shown to help improve symptoms of fibromyalgia, specifically pain.
- **Vitamin B6 (pyridoxine)** supports the central nervous system as well as metabolism. It also helps to turn food into energy and helps with the creation of neurotransmitters, such as dopamine and serotonin which works as an anti-depressant.
- **Vitamin B9 (folate acid)** helps with proper brain function as well as playing an important role in mental and emotional well-being. B9 is also instrumental in the body's genetic material.
- **Vitamin B12 (cyanocobalamin)** plays an important role in ensuring the normal function of the brain and the central nervous system.
- **Vitamin C** acts as an antioxidant, protecting your cells from damage as well as reduce physical impairment.
- **Vitamin E** can act as an antioxidant, protecting your cells from damage caused by free radicals. Vitamin E is also essential to the health of your vision, health of your blood and your immune system.
- **Calcium** helps keep muscles working properly as well as supports the central nervous system.
- **Magnesium** helps to avoid muscle spasms, weakness and back pain as well as keeping the heart, kidneys and bones healthy and strong. Getting enough magnesium can help with fatigue, sleep difficulties, and anxiety.

- **Ginger** is helpful in pain management and can ease nausea and improve digestion. Ginger can also increase antioxidant activity in the body due to its anti-inflammatory and antibacterial chemicals which are antioxidants.

Plantar Fasciitis (Heel Pain)

Plantar fasciitis is a condition which causes pain on the bottom of the heel and radiates across the arch of the foot. It occurs when the band of tissue which supports the arch of your foot becomes inflamed, causing stabbing pain.

Causes/Risk Factors

- **Sex** – women tend to get plantar fasciitis more than men
- **Obese or pregnant** – being overweight is a contributing factor as is becoming pregnant.
- **Age** – usually occurs between the ages of 40 and 70.
- **Feet condition** – having flat feet or very high arches are a contributing factor.
- **Activity** – Taking part in dancing of toes, running and jumping can lead to serious plantar fasciitis.
- **Achilles** – when you have tight Achilles tendons, you place more strain on the band of tissue under your feet.

Usual Treatments

- **Physical therapy** – Stretching and learning stretching exercises to do at home can help relieve the pressure, pain and strengthen the band tissue under the foot.

- **Massage** – helps to relieve the pain and pressure and relax the band of tissue that is inflamed in your heel and arch.
- **Medications** – some medications are prescribed for pain, inflammation, and muscle relaxation.
- **Devices** – braces and splints can be prescribed to help lend support to the affected areas.
- **Self-care** – don't forget your "RICE"! (Rest, ice, compression, elevation). Shoe inserts can be used as well as having other shoe modifications done. While it is good to continue exercising and sticking to daily activities, you may have to modify them until you have relief of your plantar fasciitis.

Healthy Alternatives

- **Vitamin B1 (thiamin)** working as an anti-inflammatory, high doses of thiamin have shown to help improve symptoms of fibromyalgia, specifically pain.
- **Vitamin B3 (niacin)** Niacin helps improve circulation, and it has been shown to suppress inflammation. Acts as natural pain reliever.
- **Vitamin B6 (pyridoxine)** helps with the creation of dopamine and serotonin which works as an anti-depressant.
- **Vitamin B12 (cyanocobalamin)** plays an important role in ensuring the normal function of the brain and the central nervous system.
- **Vitamin C** acts as an antioxidant, protecting your cells from damage as well as reduce physical impairment.
- **Vitamin D** has anti-inflammatory properties which contribute to relieving pain and may alleviate other symptoms.
- **Vitamin E** can act as an antioxidant, protecting your cells from damage caused by free radicals. Vitamin E is also

essential to the health of your vision, health of your blood and your immune system.

- **Magnesium** helps to avoid muscle spasms, weakness and back pain as well as keeping the heart, kidneys and bones healthy and strong. Getting enough magnesium can help with fatigue, sleep difficulties, and anxiety.

Other healthy alternatives

Various herbal treatments can help improve the symptoms of plantar fasciitis. Some of the most popular herbs and spices for inflammation include turmeric, tree tea, cinnamon, black pepper, and ginger. Omega-3 is also great for plantar fasciitis because it contains healthy fatty acid which can reduce inflammation and improve heel pain.

Please do not stop taking your prescribed medications like I did without consulting your care provider first.

PSORIASIS

Is an autoimmune condition which happens when skin cells multiply faster than they should and builds up on the surface of the body. Dry, thick, and raised patches on the skin are the most common sign of psoriasis. Inflammation and redness are common and typical psoriatic scales are whitish-silver and develop in thick, red patches. What appears as an itchy rash can turn into a real serious problem if you continue to scratch it.

My experience

Four years ago, I was walking and all of a sudden, I felt as though I had been stung or bitten by something on the back of my calf. The next day there was a reddish spot about the size of a quarter. I figured it would go away after a few weeks and to my surprise, it actually got bigger until it was the size of my fist and was very itchy.

I went to the doctor and was given some topical ointment to put on the area twice a day. Of course, to me, it just seemed to get all over everything and did nothing to relieve the itching and redness. This went on several years and at one point, even had a biopsy done on it.

I went to a dermatologist who I thought was whacked when she told me to soak in a tub of water with bleach in it. "Say what?"

There were other reasons why I didn't take her advice to heart but that is a story for another time. I left frustrated as well as feeling it was a waste of time.

A year and a half later, I decided to get another opinion and scheduled an appointment with a dermatologist at the VA clinic where I saw a resident doctor. We hit it off right away and I shared with him my story of this darn rash which wouldn't go away. I even told him about the whole bleach idea and he tells me there is some truth to it. Who knew but I was still not going to try it.

After examining my leg, he prescribed another topical ointment for me to apply twice a day for 2 weeks. Only this time, I was supposed to wrap my calf in saran wrap. This would keep it from getting all over everything but also, force the ointment to absorb into my skin. So, I did as I was told and I was quite impressed with how quickly it began to show signs of healing.

I was told I would see a decrease in the raised skin, the itchiness would subside and my calf would begin to feel normal again. Of course, I was told the pigmentation would take about 6 months to go back to normal but who cares, do you know how difficult it is to look back at your calves? Trust me, I couldn't see it without contorting my body.

I had more trouble with the saran wrap than I did with the ointment but I finally got the coordination down to get it wrapped. I only went out in public once with the leg wrapped in saran wrap. I certainly didn't need people looking at me and thinking I was nuts. Going across the street and hanging out with friends was a different story, they already knew I was nuts!

It didn't take long and I truly saw awesome results. My calf looked and felt so much better and I wasn't even tempted to scratch at it one time or another.

Note: Perhaps had I known about the saran wrap trick when first diagnosed with Psoriasis and prescribed the ointment, I would have gotten it under control right away and not suffered with it for almost 4 years. It took almost 4 long years to gain this one piece of information.

Note #2: While I know this isn't the section you are expecting at this time, I still need to let you know that while the Clobetasol Propionate ointment worked to clear up my psoriasis completely, I had been applying 2000 iu of vitamin D on the area for about 6 months prior and had received relief from the itching irritation. I think it was the vitamin D which saved my insanity with regards to this rash.

Now on to causes/risk factors!

Causes/Risk Factors

- **Stress** – Stress in one's life can have an adverse effect on the body in many ways and psoriasis is one of them. Whether it is being under a deadline for work or studying for an exam or even simply worrying where your next month's rent is coming from can cause your body to react, causing rashes and other autoimmune problems.
- **Genetic** – Family history is another risk factor on determining the cause. Genes are passed on from generation to generation.
- **Obesity** – carrying excess weight can contribute to psoriasis developing in the folds of the body, mainly in the areas of groin, buttocks and breasts.
- **Lifestyle** – The usual suspects such as smoking and drinking alcohol contribute to psoriasis by affecting the immune system.

- **Medications** – There are some medications which have side-effects that are consistent with the development of psoriasis.
- **Other Skin problems** – Whether it is a skin injury or perhaps a viral and/or bacterial infection, there are a number of skin ailments which can lead to psoriasis.

Usual Treatments

While Psoriasis can't be cured at this time, there are several different treatments available to lessen the severity as well as even clear up affected skin areas. Some of them are;

- **Medications** – Just turn on the television, you are bound to see a commercial for a new drug being peddled for psoriasis. Of course, there are the usual steroid creams and ointments which are prescribed like the one I mentioned, Clobetasol Propionate ointment but just beware, follow the directions closely to avoid developing other health issues.
- **Phototherapy** – Also known as photodynamic therapy where your skin is exposed to different types of ultraviolet light, killing off skin cells.
- **Self-Care** – There are a lot of ways one can help themselves when psoriasis develops. Learning to relax, become stress free and improve one's mental health can help your body in so many ways. Using moisturizers, petroleum jelly, and other natural skin care products can also help.

Healthy Alternatives

- **Vitamin A** helps with body pain as it helps your immune system and the development of new skin cells.
- **Vitamin B7 (biotin)** helps promote appropriate function of the nervous system and is essential for liver metabolism. Biotin is commonly used to strengthen hair and nails, as well as in skin care. It also aids cell growth as well as helps the maintenance of mucous membranes.
- **Vitamin B12 (cyanocobalamin)** plays an important role in ensuring the normal function of the brain and the central nervous system as well as boosts the immune system and the development of skin cells.
- **Vitamin C** acts as an antioxidant, protecting your cells from damage as well as reducing physical impairment.
- **Vitamin D** has anti-inflammatory properties which contribute to relieving pain and may alleviate other symptoms. Applying vitamin D to the affected area may help relieve the symptoms commonly associated with psoriasis such as itchiness and redness.
- **Vitamin E** can act as an antioxidant, protecting your cells from damage caused by free radicals. Vitamin E helps reduce the itching and flakiness found with psoriasis.
- **Turmeric** with incredible anti-inflammatory properties, turmeric helps to alleviate muscle pain and inflammation discomfort. Turmeric helps relieve psoriasis symptoms. Curcumin is the active ingredient in turmeric and is known to be a healing ingredient.
- **Magnesium** helps to shed off skin cell build-up and lessen the itch.

Post-Traumatic Stress Disorder (PTSD)

Post-traumatic stress disorder is a condition of persistent mental and emotional stress occurring as a result of injury or severe psychological shock, typically involving vivid recall of the experience, disturbance of sleep and with diminished responses to others and to the outside world.

My experience

There are many things which can contribute to PTSD in one's life but not everyone is aware that they have it. That was my case. It wasn't until someone else made an observation in my behavior, I did some research, and eventually saw a couple doctors, was I diagnosed with PTSD.

It all started back on December 9th, 1985, when I was 22 years old and in the military. I was part of a unit which was training national guard units on a particular military weapon.

It was a crisp, sunny morning and I was wearing my uniform with an issued field jacket. Every morning before training or any kind of maneuvers, we were required to inspect and check over the vehicle and weapons system to be sure everything was in working order.

I began my checks and inspection as required, eventually making my way up on top of the vehicle to continue my inspection of the weapons system. Like always, I am talking with other soldiers as they were doing their checks and inspections too. All of a sudden, it happened.

My anti-tank, guided missile weapon went off by itself with me standing next to it. While the loud boom was deafening, I remember the backblast flame only being a about 18 inches but yet, the heat got up to 4,000 degrees. All I could feel at the time of the blast, was the back of my hand, and my face in different places. I looked to my right and saw my field jacket on fire.

The moment I saw this, kindergarten came back to mind. The whole "Stop, Drop & Roll". The only problem was, I was on top of this track vehicle and couldn't just drop. So, I did the next best thing which was to jump off and away from the vehicle as far as I could before landing and floundering like a fish out of water on my one side.

It was said that I looked like a fireball in the sky and a dying fish flopping on the ground. Several people came to my aid and started yanking off my field jacket to get the flames out and away from me. Again, all I could think about was my face, how bad and deformed it must be.

Don't get me wrong, I wasn't being arrogant but I liked my looks and was considered a good-looking guy. I had plans for those looks too! Being the son of a professional photographer and having already been a model in a catalog, I thought that this would end a potential career before it had a chance to begin.

As they walked me up towards all the building, to get medical attention, I remember the medic running out of the side of a building, almost completely past us. When he saw my arm, he thought I was a cook and I had dumped a large kettle of boiling water on my arm. Yes, it was that bad but what about my face? Why was no one checking out my face? Was it that bad?

My one and only ambulance ride took me to an emergency room where they frantically attended to my arm. I was coming in and out of sedation and every time I did, I kept thinking, why aren't they doing anything to my face? That was where the real pain was coming from. Of course, I was happy I could see and my hearing was starting to improve as well. I could see so many medical personnel working and focusing on me. I was thinking to myself "this is crazy, how are they all fitting around me to do what they were doing?' Truly amazing!

While I know I so concerned about my face, I was grateful to be alive and to have all these people caring for me. Even today thinking about it causes me to tear up.

The next 6 weeks were going to be a chaotic time moving forward. In the hospital for 2 weeks, getting my bandages changed, getting fluids pumped into me, and enduring the debridement process. The latter was the worst experience I have ever felt. Yet, when I saw an 18-month-old boy enduring the same thing after falling and grabbing a space heater, I sucked it up!

It was looking like I was going to be spending Christmas in the hospital according to my doctor but seeing as the "floor nurse" outranked him, I was sent home for 2 weeks with strict instructions to go to the nearest military base and have them replace my burn dressing every 3 days. Yeah, that lasted a whole whopping 2 days.

I went to the military base for the dressing change and a few hours later, I was in excruciating pain. So much so, that I was taken to the urgent care of the local hospital. Once it was my time, I was taken upstairs to a treatment room because they couldn't get my dressing off to see what the problem was. By now, you can imagine what the problem actually was.

The nurse tried to remove the dressing again but knew it would cause more pain as well as damage to my arm. So, she left, came back with a doctor who examined the situation and asked questions, only to leave again and come back in with another doctor. After they examined the situation once more, they left the room.

By now I am in a lot of stress but also curious as to what was going on. The first doctor came in, talked with the nurse and then told me what was going to happen. The nurse placed my arm in a whirlpool tub to soften the dressing to allow it to be removed with the least amount of damage to my wound. They were going to dress my burn correctly but, that was not all.

The doctor had asked me how long I was in town and as I told him just under 2 weeks, he instructed me to not return to the military base for treatment but to come to the local hospital every two days for my treatment and replacement of the dressing. Since I was in the military, I was in the mode of following orders. So, I did!

It turns out when I went to the military base to get the dressing changed, they forgot one key element. They didn't apply Silvadene cream to the burn, they just put the dressing against the burn and wrapped it. This is what caused the excruciating pain.

After the 2 weeks at home, I went back and became a medical hold, meaning I was still under strict restriction but not needing to be in the hospital. However, I was supposed to show up to the hospital to do work. This lasted a week before I asked to be released back to my unit and placed on light duty for a couple weeks.

As you can see, I had two traumatic events within a short period of time which led to my post-traumatic stress disorder. A disorder I wouldn't even realize I had for another 26 years!

Causes/Risk Factors

Once again, PTSD is the mental and emotional stress occurring as a result of injury or severe psychological shock experienced in one's life. Here are some risk factors to be aware of;

- **Age** – anyone can develop PTSD at any age. This includes children.
- **Military veterans** – imagine what military personnel go through. Whether it's the intense and sometimes brutal training to the sounds and sights of being in a combat zone. Our veterans are some of the most vulnerable for having PTSD.
- **Sexual assault/abuse survivors** – some people have experienced traumatic events which have scarred them for life while others have been repeatedly traumatized from ongoing abuse.
- **Disasters victims** – losing your worldly possessions due to a tornado, hurricane, or a fire can have a lasting effect on someone.
- **Accidents** – serious accidents and other serious injuries can have an effect on one's quality of life and then lead to struggles with PTSD.
- **Genetics** – researchers continue to study the brain and how genetics plays a role in those who experience PTSD.

There are other symptoms and behaviors which can result from a traumatic experience and I am listing mine simply to give others an example of what they might experience but aren't aware it could be part of a PTSD experience for them.

When I was first diagnosis with PTSD, I was given a VA disability rating of 30%. This diagnosis was based off the following;

Occupational and social impairment with occasional decrease in work efficiency and intermittent periods of inability to perform occupational tasks (although generally functioning satisfactorily, with routine behavior, self-care, and normal conversation) due to such symptoms as: depressed mood, anxiety, suspiciousness, panic attacks (weekly or less often), chronic sleep impairment, mild memory loss (such as forgetting names, directions, recent events)

Nine years later, my VA PTSD disability rating was bumped up to 50%, based on;

Occupational and social impairment with reduced reliability and productivity due to such symptoms as: flattened affect; circumstantial, circumlocutory, or stereotyped speech; panic attacks more than once a week; difficulty in understanding complex commands; impairment of short- and long-term memory (e. g. retention of only highly learned material, forgetting to complete tasks); impaired judgment; impaired abstract thinking; disturbances of motivation and mood; difficulty in establishing and maintaining effective work and social relationships.

There are times when I do get overwhelmed working on all my projects I have going on and need to step away as I start to panic and lose all function. At least I have a good idea what triggers it and know when I am starting to feel out of control.

So, let's move on to what can be done.

Usual Treatments

Because everyone is different and experience events differently, not all treatments work for every person. In other words, what works for me, may not work for you. That's why there are several courses of treatment, including;

- **Cognitive behavioral therapy** – a type of psychotherapy which focuses on negative patterns of thought about self as well as the world and confront these negative thought patterns in order to change unwanted behavioral patterns and treat disorders such as anxiety and depression.
- **Exposure therapy** – is used to help people with PTSD cope with the feelings by helping people face and control their fears. This is done by gradually exposing them to the trauma they experienced but in a safe way. It is likened to

helping them replace a bad memory with a healthy positive one. Tools used include visiting the site of the trauma, writing about it and their feelings as well as using imagery in order to help change thought patterns and memory.

- **Cognitive restructuring** – When some people remember events differently than how they really occurred, cognitive restructuring helps them make sense of those bad memories. It is a way of looking at the event realistically without feeling guilty or ashamed of their feelings and actions.
- **Medications** – Usually antidepressants are prescribed the most with those who suffer from PTSD. Some medications help with lessening nightmares and aid sleeping.
- **Counseling** – meeting with a counselor or psychologist can help ease the symptoms of PTSD with some people. The ability to talk through the events and speak about the trauma and your feelings may benefit someone with PTSD.

Healthy Alternatives

- **Vitamin B1 (thiamin)** working as an anti-inflammatory, high doses of thiamin have shown to help improve symptoms of anxiety and inflammatory responses to trauma.
- **Vitamin B2 (riboflavin)** is a water-soluble vitamin and helps prevent headaches and visual disturbances brought on by stress and anxiety.
- **Vitamin B3 (niacin)** helps improve circulation, and it has been shown to suppress inflammation. Acts as natural pain reliever as well as helps to calm nerves to induce sleep.
- **Vitamin B5 (pantothenic acid)** helps in the manufacturing of red blood cells, maintaining healthy digestive tracts and most importantly production of anti-stress hormones. Helps build energy molecules.

- **Vitamin B6 (pyridoxine)** supports the central nervous system as well as metabolism. It also helps to turn food into energy and helps with the creation of neurotransmitters, such as dopamine and serotonin which works as an anti-depressant.
- **Vitamin B9 (folate acid)** helps with proper brain function as well as playing an important role in mental and emotional well-being. B9 is also instrumental in the body's genetic material.
- **Vitamin B12 (cyanocobalamin)** plays an important role in ensuring the normal function of the brain and the central nervous system. Helps reduce stress.
- **Vitamin C** acts as an antioxidant, protecting your cells from damage as well as reduce physical impairment. It is also water-soluble for easy absorption. May help with reducing oxidative stress and prevent memory impairment.
- **Vitamin E** can act as an antioxidant, protecting your cells from damage caused by free radicals. Vitamin E is also essential to the health of your vision, health of your blood and your immune system. Vitamin E helps prevent memory impairment.
- **Turmeric** with incredible anti-inflammatory properties, turmeric helps to alleviate muscle pain and inflammation discomfort.
- **Magnesium** Getting enough magnesium can help with fatigue, sleep difficulties, and anxiety as well as memories.
- **Ginger** can help improve memory and focus. Helps protect the brain after a brain trauma.

Please do not stop taking your prescribed medications like I did without consulting your care provider first.

RESTLESS LEG SYNDROME (RLS)

Having an irresistible need to move your legs, usually at night? It is quite certain you are experiencing restless leg syndrome. This condition can affect you whether you are sitting or lying down. It can feel as though you have creeping and crawling sensations in your legs.

Causes/Risk Factors

While the cause of RLS is still unknown, symptoms can also vary from person to person. People who experience RLS have reported the following symptoms;

- Creeping sensation
- Crawling sensation
- Throbbing sensation
- Itching sensation
- Aching sensation

Symptoms can vary in severity.

Usual Treatments

The usual treatments for RLS primarily involve medications, such as;

- **Medications** to treat neuropathy symptoms to lessen the communication between nerves. Such medications include gabapentin (Neurontin) and pregabalin (Lyrica).
- **Muscle relaxants** sometimes used in conjunction with opioids to help relax leg nerves.
- **Sleep medication** to help you sleep better but won't eliminate the creeping and crawling sensations.
- **Opioids** may relieve severe symptoms.

Healthy Alternatives

- **Vitamin A** helps with body pain as it helps your immune system, eyesight, reproduction and growth and development. It also helps the lungs, heart and other organs work properly.
- **Vitamin B12 (cyanocobalamin)** plays an important role in ensuring the normal function of the brain and the central nervous system. B12 has been directly linked to helping alleviate symptoms of RLS.
- **Vitamin C** acts as an antioxidant, protecting your cells from damage as well as reduce physical impairment.
- **Vitamin D** has anti-inflammatory properties which contribute to relieving pain and may alleviate other symptoms. Studies have found vitamin D helps reduce RLS symptoms.
- **Vitamin E** can act as an antioxidant, protecting your cells from damage caused by free radicals.

- **Turmeric** with incredible anti-inflammatory properties, turmeric helps to alleviate muscle pain and inflammation discomfort.
- **Magnesium** helps to avoid muscle spasms, weakness and back pain as well as keeping the heart, kidneys and bones healthy and strong. Getting enough magnesium can help with fatigue, sleep difficulties, and anxiety.

SHINGLES
(VARICELLA ZOSTER VIRUS)

Is a painful rash on the body caused by the reactivation of the chickenpox virus in the body. Anyone who has had chickenpox in their lifetime may develop shingles.

This type of rash appears as a large strip of blister like sores. While the rash normally shows up on the trunk of the body, some people have experienced it as a cold sore by their mouth or even experienced it around their eyes, which can be very dangerous. Pain can persist even after the rash is gone; this is called postherpetic neuralgia.

Causes/Risk Factors

While there is no known cause which reactivates the virus, here are the common risk factors:

- **Age** – Shingle outbreaks most commonly occur in adults over 50.
- **Chronic medical condition** – such as diabetes, cancer (leukemia and lymphoma)

- **HIV (human immunodeficiency virus)** – people with HIV can have multiple occurrences of shingles while it usually happens a singular time with non-HIV patients.
- **Organ transplant** – medications used to suppress the immune system to prevent the rejection of the organ.

Usual Treatments

It is said that the shingles virus can and will go away on its own, it could take up to 4 weeks. Medications are available to accelerate the healing process such as creams. Other medication might be prescribed for the pain and anxiety.

Healthy Alternatives

- **Vitamin A** helps with body pain as it helps your immune system, eyesight, and helps with body wound healing.
- **Vitamin B12 (cyanocobalamin)** plays an important role in ensuring the normal function of the brain and the central nervous system.
- **Vitamin C** acts as an antioxidant, protecting your cells from damage as well as reducing physical impairment. It also helps with nerve pain of shingles after the rash has healed.
- **Vitamin D** has anti-inflammatory properties which contribute to relieving pain and may alleviate other symptoms. Also increases immune response and lowers inflammation.
- **Vitamin E** can act as an antioxidant, protecting your cells from damage caused by free radicals. Vitamin E is also essential to the health of your vision, health of your blood and your immune system.

- **Turmeric** eases the pain of post-shingles nerve irritation.
- **Zinc** used to prevent the virus from spreading and inhibit recurrences.

Sleep Apnea

Sleep Apnea is a medical condition where you repeatedly stop and start breathing while you sleep. There are several types of sleep apnea;

1. Obstructive sleep apnea (OSA), the most common, is caused by a blockage of the airway during sleep. In obstructive sleep apnea, throat muscles relax and a person's tongue and soft palate collapse against the back of the throat during sleep, closing the airway and causing snoring.
2. Central sleep apnea (CSA), is caused by the brain failing to send the right signals to the muscles which control breathing during sleep. There is no airway blockage in CSA and is quite rare.
3. Mixed sleep apnea (AKA Complex sleep apnea syndrome), as the name implies, is a combination of both OSA and CSA.

Causes/Risk Factors

The risk factors of both obstructive and central sleep apneas overlap, making it difficult to determine which type you have. The most common signs and symptoms of obstructive and central sleep apneas may include;

- Loud snoring
- Gasping for air during sleep
- Stopping and starting breathing while sleeping
- Bad breath due to dry mouth
- Difficulty staying asleep
- Excessive daytime drowsiness
- Headaches in the morning
- Irritability

Other symptoms of concern caused by the stopping and starting of breathing while sleeping;

- Depression
- High blood pressure
- Heart disease
- Stroke
- Diabetes

Usual Treatments

- **Diagnosis** – If you are experiencing any of the above symptoms, you should see your doctor to discuss diagnosis as well as course of action.
- **CPAP Therapy** – stands for Continuous Positive Air Pressure (CPAP) machine. This machine sits by the bed with a plastic hose connected to a face mask. You wear the face mask while you sleep. The CPAP delivers constant steady air flow to help you breath while sleeping. A CPAP machine recipient must complete a sleep study prior to delivery of machine.
- **Sleep study** – There are two types of sleep studies which can be performed. In-Clinic sleep study and At-home sleep

study. These studies are completed during your normal sleep pattern.

1. In-clinic sleep study – you spend a night at a clinic where they observe and record your sleep habits as well as record your breathing habits while sleeping. Equipment is in clinic.
2. At-home sleep study – you get to do the sleep study in the comfort of your own home and bed. The equipment will be delivered to your home and will do just as it does with the in-clinic sleep study. Measure your breathing as well as monitor your sleep habits.

- **Lifestyle changes** – Losing weight, eating health foods
- **Behavioral changes** – learning to sleep on your side instead of your back.

Note: Probably should have put the in-home sleep study first because depending on the results of the in-home study, you may then be required to do an in-hospital sleep study.

Healthy Alternatives

- **Vitamin B12 (cyanocobalamin)** plays an important role in ensuring the normal function of the brain and the central nervous system.
- **Vitamin C** can reduce the number of apnea episodes in the night and also improve sleep quality which can reduce the amount of daytime sleepiness.
- **Vitamin D** has anti-inflammatory properties which contribute to relieving pain and may alleviate other symptoms, helping to promote quality sleep and helps lessen snoring as well as other sleep disorders.
- **Vitamin E** can reduce the number of apnea episodes in the night and also improve sleep quality which can reduce the

amount of daytime sleepiness. Vitamin E is also essential to the health of your vision, health of your blood and your immune system.

- **Vitamin K2** allows deep, restorative sleep so the brain can heal.
- **Magnesium** getting enough magnesium can help with fatigue, sleep difficulties, and anxiety as it works to keep the brain and body calm.
- **Ginger** acts as an anti-inflammatory and antibacterial agent and increases saliva secretion, which soothes the throat and provides relief from snoring.

TENDINITIS

Tendinitis (also called tendonitis) is an inflammation or irritation of a tendon, a thick cord which attaches bone to muscle. Have you ever heard of tennis elbow? Now you know what tendinitis is and trust me, it can be very painful and annoying.

Causes/Risk Factors

While pain is the primary symptom, there are other symptoms and conditions to be aware of. Such as;

- **Achilles tendinitis** – an injury or irritation of the tendon which connects the calf muscle to the heel bone. People who operate riding lawn mowers will experience this sort of irritation after hours of pushing down on the forward/reverse drive.
- **Swimmer's shoulder** – shoulder pain after repetitive motion due to a tendon (connective tissue) rubbing on the shoulder blade.
- **Golfer's elbow** – the same as tennis elbow but different as the pain is usually on the inside of the elbow as opposed to the outside for tennis elbow.
- **Jumper's knee** – an injury to the patellar tendon which connects the kneecap to the shin bone.

- **De Quervain's tenosynovitis** – a painful condition affecting the tendons on the thumb side of the wrists.
- **Tendinitis of the wrist** – swelling of the tendons connecting muscle to bones in the wrist.

Usual Treatments

- **Achilles tendinitis** – at home rest, icing, and pain relievers with a doctor's supervision.
- **Swimmer's shoulder** – medication, rest and relaxation as well as physical therapy.
- **Golfer's elbow** – treatment includes at-home rest, icing, pain relievers, stretching and/or physical therapy, and elbow brace.
- **Tennis elbow** – treatment includes at-home rest, icing, pain relievers, stretching and/or physical therapy, and elbow brace.
- **Jumper's knee** – treatment usually consists of pain relief measures and physical therapy
- **De Quervain's tenosynovitis** – treatment includes medication, physical therapy and possible surgery.
- **Tendinitis of the wrist** – mostly at-home rest, icing, pain relievers, physical therapy, and sometimes steroids are injected into the tendon.

Healthy Alternatives

- **Vitamin A** is important for cell division, collagen renewal, tissue repair, and vision. Vitamin A increases the elasticity of collagen, maintaining strength of tendons and ligaments.
- **Vitamin C** acts as an antioxidant, protecting your cells from damage as well as reducing physical impairment. Vitamin C positively affects tendon healing by helping to increase

the collagen fibril diameter and the number of fibroblasts at the injured area.

- **Vitamin D** has anti-inflammatory properties which contribute to relieving pain and may alleviate other symptoms.
- **Vitamin E** can act as an antioxidant, protecting your cells from damage caused by free radicals. Vitamin E is also essential to the health of your vision, health of your blood and your immune system.
- **Turmeric (curcumin)** with incredible anti-inflammatory properties, turmeric helps to alleviate muscle pain and inflammation discomfort.
- **Omega 3 (EPA & DHA)** has positive effects on inflammation, decreasing oxidative stress, and supports post-workout recovery.
- **Magnesium** aids the healing of connective tissues and muscles.
- **Calcium** also aids the healing of connective tissues and muscles.
- **Ginger** is helpful in pain management and can ease nausea and improve digestion. Ginger can also increase antioxidant activity in the body due to its anti-inflammatory and antibacterial chemicals which are antioxidants.

Please do not stop taking your prescribed medications like I did without consulting your care provider first.

TINNITUS (RINGING IN THE EAR)

While tinnitus is not a disease in itself, it is still an ailment which is seen as a symptom of an underlying issue with the body's auditory system. This includes the ear, the auditory nerve, the brain and the parts of the brain which process sound. Those underlying conditions could be;

- Migraines
- Anemia
- Thyroid issues
- Diabetes
- Autoimmune disorders

Causes/Risk Factors

- **Age** – age-related hearing loss comes on gradually as we age.
- **Exposure to loud noises** – whether you are at a concert, worked on a loud construction site, or been to a noisy airport, you have experienced some hearing loss. Most times, your hearing is gradually restored but over time, the recovery process can take longer.
- **Earwax build-up** – as crazy as it sounds, earwax build up is a major culprit in the hearing loss of children.

- **Abnormal bone growth in ear** – another common cause of hearing loss in young adults. The three tiny bones in the ear which contribute to vibrations when sound waves enter.
- **Head & neck injuries** – injuries can damage any one of these critical parts of the ear including: rupture in the eardrum, damage to the ossicles and/or hair cells, restricted blood flow, and obstructed auditory pathways.
- **Stress and depression** when you are stressed or depressed, the overproduction of adrenaline reduces blood flow to the ears, affecting hearing.
- **Water in ear** – when water accumulates in the ear and doesn't drain properly, you risk developing swimmer's ear, or another type of infection which can cause hearing loss if not treated.

Diagnosis Methods

- **Physical examination** – healthcare provider will check your ears for any obvious problems.
- **Hearing test** – this test checks your ability to hear a range of tones, displaying your results in an audiogram.

Usual Treatments

- **Hearing aids** – Many people who have tinnitus also have hearing aids to help provide relief from tinnitus by making sounds louder and the tinnitus less noticeable.
- **Medications** – are provided for any pain related to tinnitus.
- **Relaxation techniques** – the stress and frustration of tinnitus can make it even more noticeable. Learning relaxation techniques can put you and your mind at ease, maybe even decrease the tinnitus level in your ears.

- **Counseling** – mental wellness therapies like cognitive behavioral therapy (CBT) or acceptance and commitment therapy (ACT) can help people learn how to pay less attention to tinnitus.

Note: With this next statement, I am not trying to offend anyone who has or is dealing with tinnitus. With that said, I am going to say "it's all in your head!", seriously! No pun intended but it is true! Well, at least for me anyway!

You see, I have been diagnosed with tinnitus and I have experienced what I call, a bug zapper sound in my ear/head. Yes, when it occurs, it is very distracting and annoying. I used to dig in my ear and even pound on my ear (not recommended) to alleviate the crackling sound. It drove me crazy!

I know, my tinnitus was brought on because I have been a drummer since I was 10 years old and I like loud music, both playing and listening to it. I was also surrounded by tanks, armored personnel carriers, and helicopters while in the military and the loud sounds of weaponry going off. Yes, we had ear plugs but they weren't very good and well, they were easily lost.

So, how did I help myself alleviate the crackling and zapping in my ear/head? I simply told it to **STOP!** That's right, I told it to **STOP! And the crazy thing is, it did!**

We all know how the mind can play tricks on us, which is what I thought it was at first too, but then when it happened again the following spring, I did it again! I told it to **STOP!** And it did!

I do have some dull hearing loss and after taking a hearing test, I know it is the 3000s and 6000s which I have an especially hard time hearing. The funny thing is, most women's voices are in the 3000s and 6000s range! I kid you not! So, ladies, I am not ignoring you, I just can't hear you at times! **Honest!**

Of course, I also take vitamins to help in all areas of my hearing and overall health!

Healthy Alternatives

- **Vitamin B9 (folate acid)** helps in preventing hearing loss and the lack of adequate folate levels seems to affect high-frequency hearing.
- **Vitamin B12 (cobalamin)** plays an important role in ensuring the normal function of the brain and the central nervous system. Studies have shown that B12 deficiency is linked to chronic hearing loss.
- **Vitamin D** has anti-inflammatory properties which contribute to relieving pain and may alleviate other symptoms such as hearing loss and ringing in the ears.
- **Magnesium** is an important ear health mineral which helps block the activity of cell-damaging molecules.
- **Potassium** – helps relax the pressure within the blood vessels as well as the fluid in our inner ear needs potassium as part of the process of converting sound into nerve impulses which get sent to the brain.
- **Zinc** is key to helping the body fight off viruses and bacteria

Please do not stop taking your prescribed medications like I did without consulting your care provider first.

THYROID DISEASE

Your thyroid gland is located in the neck, just above your collarbone. It's one of your endocrine system glands, which make hormones. Thyroid disease is when your thyroid has one of three issues and they are;

Hyperthyroidism (overactive thyroid) – a condition where your thyroid gland produces too much of the hormone thyroxine. Hyperthyroidism can cause your metabolism to speed up which then causes a variety of concerns and symptoms, including:

- Nervousness, anxiety, and irritability
- Tremors in hands and fingers
- Sweating
- Sudden weight loss
- Increase sensitivity to heat
- Fatigue, muscle weakness
- Menstrual pattern changes
- Hair becomes fine and brittle
- Bowel movement changes
- An enlarged thyroid gland
- Thinning skin

Hypothyroidism (underactive thyroid) – a condition where your thyroid gland doesn't produce enough thyroid hormone and disturbs the normal balance of chemical reactions in your body, mainly in your metabolism, which slows. Depending on the severity of the hormone deficiency, symptoms can vary. Symptoms of hypothyroidism include:

- Constipation
- Fatigue
- Weight gain
- Puffy face
- Dry skin
- Sensitivity to cold
- Slowed heart rate
- Memory loss
- Depression
- Pain
- Irregular menstrual cycle
- Stiff & swollen joints

Thyroid nodules – are solid or liquid-filled lumps which form within the thyroid gland. These nodules aren't considered serious and don't have any symptoms. In fact, most people don't even know they have them until they are discovered during a medical exam.

Usual Treatments

Hyperthyroidism (overactive thyroid)

Medications – are used to stop the thyroid from producing excess hormones. The main types used are carbimazole and propylthiouracil.

Radioactive iodine – taken by mouth and is absorbed by the thyroid, causing it to shrink and destroy the thyroid tissue.

Surgery – thyroidectomy is when a major portion of the thyroid gland is removed.

Hypothyroidism (underactive thyroid)

Medications – such as synthetic thyroid hormone levothyroxine (Levoxyl, Synthroid,) to restore adequate levels.

Healthy Alternatives

- **Vitamin A** has been shown to help regulate thyroid hormone metabolism and inhibit thyroid-stimulating hormone (TSH) secretion.
- **Vitamin B3 (niacin)** it is thought that vitamin B3 may decrease thyroid hormone levels.
- **Vitamin B12 (cyanocobalamin)** plays a role in red cell metabolism. It also increases your energy and strengthens your nervous system.
- **Vitamin C** is vital for your thyroid and body to stay healthy! Is required for biosynthesis of collagen, protein metabolism and functions as an antioxidant to strengthen the immune system to prevent infections, cold and flu.
- **Vitamin D** improved TSH levels in subjects with hypothyroidism as well as thyroid antibodies in people with autoimmune thyroiditis.
- **Vitamin E** improves hypothyroid symptoms through its antioxidant effects.
- **Turmeric(curcumin)** shows tumor-inhibiting activity in thyroid cancer. Curcumin may protect against the genetic

damage and side effects induced by radioactive iodine, a known treatment.

- **Ginger** is known to have antioxidative properties along with control on metabolic rate and inflammation, which helps to keep thyroid hormones in control.
- **Zinc** is needed for thyroid hormone production and is key to helping the body fight off viruses and bacteria.
- **Iodine** is an important element for production of thyroid hormones. Since the body does not produce iodine, it is an essential part of anyone's diet.

Please do not stop taking your prescribed medications like I did without consulting your care provider first.

CONCLUSION

In this book, I only mentioned the 25 ailments which I have either experienced myself or know someone else who has or is experiencing it. Did you know there are around 150 most common diagnosis ailments in the U.S.? So, this is just a sample of those.

While I wrote about the 25 in this book, my team and I plan to create webinars on so many others too.

We may start a podcast about ailments and how vitamins and supplements can benefit you.

The point is, there is so much information out there about ailments and alternatives. I could name several entities which are a wealth of medical knowledge when it comes to ailments and their treatment. Unfortunately, if you want to know what vitamins, minerals, and supplements can be used as an alternative, you have to put in the work to discover for yourself.

While the vitamin and supplement market size was USD 119.66 billion in 2020, this industry still gets a bad rap due to scrupulous individuals. The vitamin and supplement industry isn't as regulated as the pharmaceutical industry is but for good reason when you consider how many new drugs come on to the market every year.

Do your homework and know what you are buying to put in your body. Be sure it is manufactured in the U.S. and in an FDA certified lab and that the products are GMO free! You owe it to yourself.

In conclusion, I hope you found value from this book. An ailment which resonates with you but also gives you the confidence to try a natural remedy to the ailment you or a loved one is dealing with.

Thank you for allowing me to have a bit of your time. I appreciate it.

I wish you well,
Frank Auenson

APPENDIX A

Vitamins & supplements discussed in book;

- **Vitamin A helps with body pain as it helps your immune system and the development of new skin cells.**
- **Vitamin B1 (thiamin)** works to help metabolize carbohydrates, fats, and proteins, activating stored energy instead of letting it turn to fat.
- **Vitamin B3 (niacin)** helps the body make various sex and stress-related hormones in the adrenal glands and other parts of the body. Niacin helps improve circulation, and it has been shown to suppress inflammation. Acts as natural pain reliever.
- **Potassium** – helps relax the pressure within the blood vessels as well as helping to lower sodium levels which can help reduce blood pressure.
- **Vitamin B5 (pantothenic acid)** helps in the manufacturing of red blood cells, maintaining healthy digestive tracts and most importantly production of anti-stress hormones. Helps build energy molecules.
- **Vitamin B6 (pyridoxine)** supports the central nervous system as well as metabolism. It also helps to turn food into energy and helps with the creation of neurotransmitters,

such as dopamine and serotonin which works as an anti-depressant.

- **Vitamin B9 (folate acid)** helps with proper brain function as well as playing an important role in mental and emotional well-being. B9 is also instrumental in the body's genetic material.
- **Vitamin B12 (cyanocobalamin)** plays an important role in ensuring the normal function of the brain and the central nervous system.
- **Vitamin C** acts as an antioxidant, protecting your cells from damage as well as reducing physical impairment.
- **Vitamin D** has anti-inflammatory properties which contribute to relieving pain and may alleviate other symptoms.
- **Calcium** is an important mineral which women need more of as estrogen levels decline. Also helps keep muscles working properly as well as supports the central nervous system.
- **CoQ10** alleviates pain and reduces brain activity and mitochondrial dysfunction. Is also able to reduce pain and increase cognition and mood in fibromyalgia.
- **Magnesium** is an important ear health mineral which helps block the activity of cell-damaging molecules.
- **Iron** is an important mineral which can help with weight loss by helping to deliver oxygen to muscles, which helps them to function. It also helps with muscle growth. Lack of iron can create low-energy and weakness.
- **Green tea** – Caffeine and catechins in green tea and other products may help with weight management.
- **Resveratrol** – This compound, found in the skin of red grapes, mulberries, peanuts, and more, may help burn fat. It thins the blood and keeps blood pressure in check. It might slow blood clotting as well. Resveratrol helps reduce

low-density lipoprotein (LDL) cholesterol (the "bad" cholesterol) and potentially help prevent damage to blood vessels. Helps with blood circulation.

- **Capsaicin** – fire up your metabolism with spicy treats to burn up to 50 extra calories per day.
- **Turmeric** – Curcumin, a compound in turmeric, is an antioxidant renowned for its anti-inflammatory properties and ability to boost metabolism. Turmeric also helps maintain brain function, fight chronic illnesses from cancer to heart disease, and much more.
- **Potassium** – helps relax the pressure within the blood vessels as well as the fluid in our inner ear needs potassium as part of the process of converting sound into nerve impulses which get sent to the brain.
- **Zinc** is key to helping the body fight off viruses and bacteria

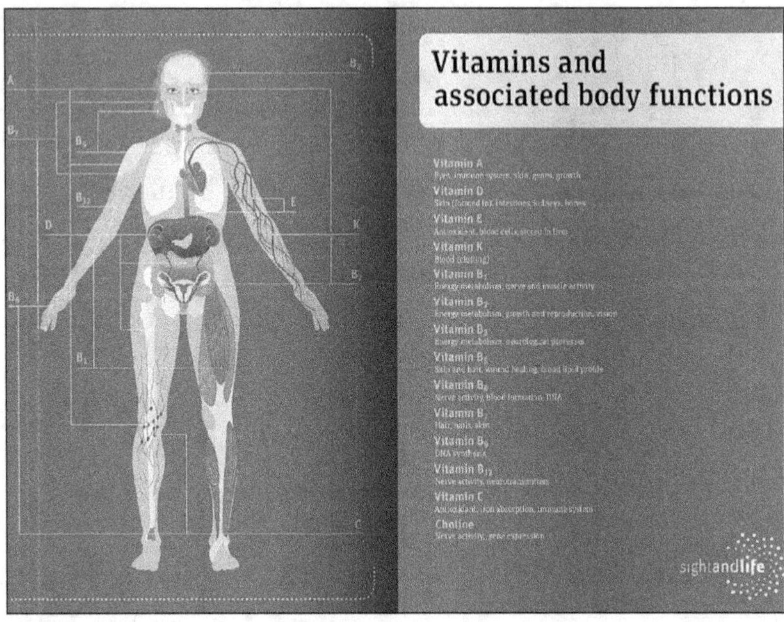

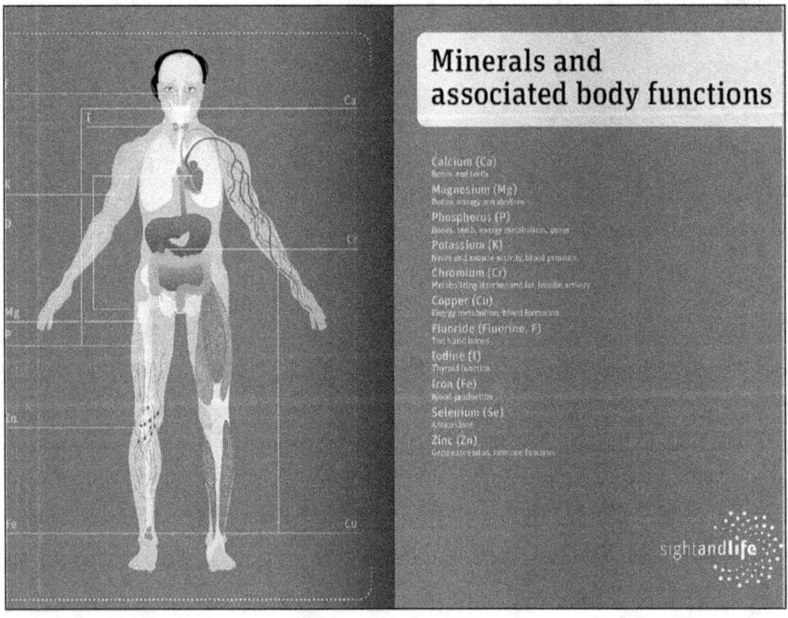

Courtesy of BioAnalyt

About the Author

Frank C Auenson

I was born Francis Adrian Swann in Madison, WI, to a woman who was 16 and in the Juvenile Center at the time. She was originally from Milwaukee and it was there that I was given up as a ward of the state because her guardian/husband to be wouldn't raise me as his own and said he would have made my life a living hell.

I proceeded to move from home to home until I was five and a half years old. I was told, one family couldn't afford to raise me, another had children that often tied me up in the attic and went downstairs to have orange juice. This happened once on a day when a social worker showed up and discovered me this way ... needless to say, I didn't finish the day staying there. I was then put into a foster home and loved it. I instantly had a big brother and older sisters who adored me. Their friends liked me too, so it was cool.

A year later, a family came to visit and took me camping. It was ok even though I did try walking away once. A few days later, the social worker came to ask if I wanted to go live with these people in Minnesota. Here is where my life got interesting. Because of what I had already experienced in my first 5 1/2 years of life, I said yes, figuring I would go live with them for a year, year and a half and then go live with someone else. It was what I knew.

What is interesting about this is that at the age of five and a half, I was given an opportunity to make a choice that was life altering. How many children under the age of six do you know that have either the opportunity or the ability to make that kind of choice? While my logic was that of a five and ½ year old, it was nonetheless a life altering decision.

Then another life altering choice was about to be presented to me in an adoption court hearing. I was asked if I wanted to change my name, and I said yes, I wanted to change it to 'Bobo', in reference to one of my foster brother's friend's nickname! This was one choice that was not allowed and now I am thankful for that! As it turned out, I never moved again and stayed with my newly adopted family for 14 years before venturing out on my own.

As I was growing up, I had many dreams and ideas of what I wanted to do with my life. I wanted to write and play music, become a real estate agent, or a recording engineer, as well as so many other possibilities, that never came true because of choices made.

While a junior in high school, I made choices without thinking of the consequences. My thought process was: "it couldn't happen to me," but I was so wrong! I became a young father during my senior year of high school. It was at that time that I was forced to do what I needed to do and forget about doing what I wanted to do.

The next 20 years found me all over the board. Jumping from job to job and thinking I had to be loved by many to feel loved. Again, bad choices dictated my life. It went from trouble with child support, to marital problems, to eventual legal troubles. It was at this time; I knew things had to change. From that moment, I chose to stay at the same job and try to 'right' my life. While I was still doing what I needed to do, thoughts of doing what I wanted to do from earlier in my life started presenting themselves to me again.

In August of 2009, I was challenged to look within myself and bring back the guy I once was and always knew I could be. I needed to ignite the flame that once drove me, and to go after my dreams even 25 years later.

What is interesting is that while I wasn't fulfilling my dreams, a friend of mine, who had no ambitions to do anything other than work in a pharmacy, became a telecommunications manager with more than 600 people under them because of the concepts and principles I instilled in them long ago. I was always telling others to go after their dreams and telling them that nothing can keep them from what they want if they truly want it. If you are willing to put the work in to achieve what you want, you can do or be anything! I was their life/success coach without even realizing it!

I have a quote that I came up with that I tell people all the time and that is "Life is what you choose it to be. It is up to you to go out and achieve. Let go of yesterday and move forward today!"

It is my wish that you see the potential that lies within you and that a spark will light the flame that drives you into becoming who you truly want to be and fulfill the dreams that you once thought were lost.

Like someone very special to me once said "Hey Bobo, you have to start some place, just start!" And start I did ...

As the "Let Me Be Frank" guy and a conscious behaviors coach, my passion is finding ways of helping people realize their dreams and challenge them to strive to bring out their potential to the fullest. I help them to get unstuck and out of their own way to get what they want in life.

I believe it starts with having higher-level thinking when it comes to decision making and choices and choosing better conscious behaviors for better living.

I won't always be politically correct, I can and will tell you "what the score is" and what I see in you. I will challenge your mind and help you design an action plan to live your life to the fullest. It's all about you discovering and believing in yourself. If you don't believe in yourself after spending time with me and your confidence isn't at a higher level, then you aren't living.

I am the coach that will push you that little bit further than you thought you could go, and then surprise you with what you can achieve! I will celebrate your accomplishments with you. I will make you laugh, and I might even make you cry, but you will be stronger and more in control of yourself and life when we reach your goals.

Allow me to motivate you!

Challenge you!

Reward you!

Believe in you!

Are you up to the challenge?

You have to start some place, so let's get started!

Connect and work with author

If you are interested in working with Frank Auenson and/or want to connect with him, see the links below:

frank@standalonefitness.com

www.standalonefitness.com

Facebook – https://www.facebook.com/Stand-Alone-Fitness-llc-106903598265696

LinkedIn – https://www.linkedin.com/in/frankauenson/

Twitter – https://twitter.com/FrankInitiative

Instagram – https://www.instagram.com/frankinitiatives/

Pinterest – https://www.pinterest.com/fauenson/

www.ingramcontent.com/pod-product-compliance
Lightning Source LLC
Chambersburg PA
CBHW070119260726
48658CB00001B/170